YOUR
MEDICINE CHEST

YOUR MEDICINE CHEST

A Consumer's Guide to Prescription and Non-Prescription Drugs

Wayne O. Evans, Ph. D.

Jonathan O. Cole, M.D.

LITTLE, BROWN AND COMPANY   BOSTON–TORONTO

FIRST EDITION

т08/78

LIBRARY OF CONGRESS CATALOGING IN PUBLICATION DATA

Evans, Wayne O.   1931–
    Your medicine chest.

    Bibliography: p.
    Includes index.
    1. Drugs. 2. Drugs, Nonprescription. I. Cole, Jonathan O.,
joint author. II. Title. [DNLM: 1. Drugs — Popular works.
2. Pharmacology — Popular works. QV38.3 E92y]
RM300.E9   615′.7   78–7497
ISBN 0–316–25823–7

Designed by Janis Capone

*Published simultaneously in Canada
by Little, Brown & Company (Canada) Limited*

PRINTED IN THE UNITED STATES OF AMERICA

To the Health of the People

Contents

YOUR
MEDICINE CHEST

Introduction

The purpose of this book is to explain the way that commonly used medicines work in your body. It tells the benefits that you can expect from the correct use of medicines and also their potential for harm. It emphasizes what you need to know to be able to ask your physician and pharmacist intelligent questions about your medicines so that you can take them safely and effectively.

There is a good deal of misinformation about drugs and their use in our society. The various forms of mass media are constantly bombarding us all with articles, advertising, and programs about drugs, both pro and con. It has become difficult for anyone, even health professionals, to keep a balanced, judicious viewpoint in the face of this deluge of information. Much of this information is biased, misleading, and in some cases, just plain untrue. Considering this, it is not surprising that some people have come to consider all drugs as evil, barely to be tolerated, and others that drugs are the wonder of modern medicine. Neither extreme is correct. For every drug there is a potential for benefit and a potential for harm that must be considered. However, knowing how the drugs work in your body, how to take them correctly, and the questions to ask your health care professional will allow you to maximize the potential benefits and minimize the potential harm.

This book reflects the conservative viewpoint of the authors. We have both spent the majority of our adult lives studying and executing research in pharmacology, that is, the study of the mechanisms of drug action. We have seen far too many excessive claims made for new drugs that were refuted when new evidence was acquired to be other than careful in the material we present. Thus, the book only discusses well-established drugs that are in common use. We have deliberately avoided drugs used in extreme medical conditions or drugs that are too new to be discussed with confidence. Our approach in discussing these drugs reflects a conservative, cautious opinion about the benefits of any of the drugs and a serious concern about potential ill effects they might produce. By the way, for the rest of the book, instead of using the term "we" to mean the authors, we shall use "I."

The principles of pharmacology explained in this book are the same as those used in the education of any health care professional. The only changes made have been in the detail in which they are explained and in the elimination of technical jargon. It is my contention that we all need to understand how drugs work in our bodies so we can take better care of ourselves. By eliminating some of the details and the jargon, the principles of pharmacology should be easily understandable to a person who has no technical training. Understanding these principles will not make you an expert in the area. You will not be able to prescribe for yourself or others. It will help in your dialogue with your physician and pharmacist about your illness and your medications.

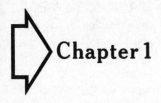

Chapter 1

What Is a Drug?

"Drug." What does that word mean to you? Do you immediately associate the term with marijuana, heroin, or other illegal chemicals? Do you think of a drug as some chemical that someone else might take, but you never would? On the other hand, think of the term "medicine." What does that word remind you of? Perhaps you think of antibiotics or other prescription compounds given to you by your physician or pharmacist. Perhaps you may even think in terms of operating rooms, white gowned surgeons, and the alien, sterile, antiseptic hush of the hospital. Consider some other terms. How about "poison," "tonic," "painkiller," "ointment," "lotion," or even "pollutant"? What kinds of images do these words bring forth in your mind? Do the words "intoxicant," "drink," "cosmetic" bring even different pictures before your eyes? They probably do. I know that, to a large extent, they do for me too. And yet, when I really think about it, I know that all these terms refer to one basic definition. They are all chemicals, of one type or another, which I ingest, have given to me, or rub on some part of my body. I expect all of these chemicals to do something to my body, whether it's to color my hair, cure a disease, or make me feel better. The common denominator for all these chemicals is the definition of the word "drug." A drug is any chemical that you place on your body, ingest, inhale, take by suppository or needle, that causes some biological change in you.

When you think about it this way you can see that we all take drugs. Almost every day we take a chemical for the purpose of changing ourselves in some way biologically. We get up in the morning and drink a cup of coffee, tea, cocoa, or perhaps a Coke. We certainly don't drink these beverages because of their nutritional value. We drink them because they make us feel better, they wake us up. They're drugs. Specifically, they are drugs that will affect our minds to make us more alert. During the day, about one in three of us will take a prescribed drug to alter the way we feel or the way our bodies function. Perhaps we will take a cold remedy or an antihistamine. Maybe it will be a tranquilizer or an antibiotic. Thinking further, even the air we breathe and the water we drink have chemicals in them. These chemicals may cause changes in our biology. Perhaps it's the sulfur dioxide in the air; we may smoke cigarettes, which load our bodies with nicotine, tars, and carbon monoxide. Later in the day, if we get a headache, have a backache, or other pain, we undoubtedly will rush to the medicine cabinet and, from the vast collection of pills of one sort or another that might be on hand, pick out an aspirin or other pain-reducing remedy. Toward evening, if we are one of the millions of Americans who drink, we will have some alcohol to relax and feel better. Or, if we're under thirty, possibly we will blow some pot to lubricate our social interactions at a party. As we go to bed, we are still not free of drugs. A good many of us will take sleeping pills, either a "non-habit-forming" type or a prescribed compound given to us by our physician. All this discussion is to try to make one point: we are surrounded by drugs.

The American people spend eleven billion dollars a year on non-prescription drugs obtained over the counter in a local drugstore or supermarket and on prescription items that we receive from a pharmacist or physician. This eleven billion dollars does not even take into account the lotions we place upon our bodies to make them prettier, upon our hair to revive, revitalize, or recolor it, or the fantastic quantities of alcohol, nicotine, and caffeinated beverages that we consume every year. Whether we like to think of ourselves this way or not, the truth of the matter is, we are a nation of drug users. Few, if any of us, get through an entire day without deliberately ingesting chemicals that will change our biological functioning in some manner.

Not only do we take drugs, but we lack knowledge about the way they act. We're really not to be blamed for our lack of knowledge. I can think of no single topic, with perhaps the exception of sex, which is so talked about and, also, so distorted with misinformation. Consider the advertising of drugs. Think about the various television programs that advertise drugs in one way or another, either through commercials or, quite often, in the actual conduct of the so-called entertainment part of the program. It's almost impossible to turn on a television set without watching the little "B's" beat the little "A's" out of the stomach, finding out about a headache compound having "twice as much of the ingredient doctors recommend most," or hearing a very serious man in a business suit telling us that we really ought to be "regular." Magazines, not only in ads, but in many of the articles, seem to have at least a third of their contents devoted to the subject of one drug or another. The new miracle cure for this, the new terror of that, or how to make ourselves healthier, happier, lovelier, and better in three easy applications of some chemical. To confuse the matter even further, we have negative drug advertising being carried on in the United States with an overwhelming zeal at the present time. This negative advertising seems to have about the same general approach and, probably, about the same accuracy, as the pro-drug advertising. It is almost impossible to escape lectures, admonitions, horror stories, and so on, about the tremendous dangers of drugs. Indeed, it has gotten to the point that many patients, when talking to their physicians, don't ask whether a drug will cure them, but ask whether it's "addicting."

Most drugs have more than one name. First, every drug has a "chemical" name. This is a long series of numbers and words that almost nobody can understand or recognize. This chemical name is probably of little interest to anyone except a medicinal chemist. Second, a drug has a "generic" name. This is the name most used by those of us who study drugs, pharmacologists. It is the name on the label of a drug that we buy at the pharmacy or supermarket. Note, however, that the "generic" name is always in very small print in a place where it is almost impossible to find. Third, there is the proprietary, or trade, name. In this book, I shall use, for the most part, the generic names of drugs. I'll also list, in parentheses, the proprietary name of some of the drugs. Some drugs have hundreds of different trade names, but each has only one generic name. Every manufacturer can give a drug his own particular trade name, and this is one problem with the use of proprietary names. We can buy the same drug under many different trade names, each at a different price. Finally, some illegal drugs have nicknames, or "street" names, slang terms assigned by their users.

I will give an example of each of the types of names, omitting the chemical name in this illustration because it is of little use and would only cause confusion. Take the sleeping pill, which is often prescribed by physicians for insomnia. One of the most common sleeping pills is a drug known by the generic name of pentobarbital. This same drug, if bought in this country, and if not in combination with something else, could be referred to as Nembutal®,* one of the proprietary names of pentobarbital, given to it by one particular manufacturing company. The nickname, or "street name," of this drug would be "yellow jacket" because pentobarbital in the form

---

* The symbol ® as a superscript indicates a proprietary name for a drug. In this book all proprietary names will have their first letter capitalized and most will be in parentheses following their generic name. The Appendix provides a list of trade and generic names of many common drugs.

generally found in this country is a 100-mg dose in a small, yellow capsule. This illustration demonstrates part of the problem that we have in discussing drugs, that is, using a different name for the same chemical. Many people have taken pentobarbital. I wonder how many would realize that they could have obtained the same drug under its generic name in the pharmacy, possibly at a lower price, if the physician had written on the prescription "pentobarbital" instead of its trade name, Nembutal. Further, I wonder how many people, when they've heard lectures on drug abuse, would ever associate the term "yellow jacket," or "downer," with the pill that may be taken, on occasion, to help get to sleep. Yet, the names in this example are all the same chemical, the same drug.

An advantage of knowing the generic names of drugs is in getting them more cheaply. Recently, I compared the prices of two non-prescription sleeping pills. The nationally advertised brand was $1.25 for 18 capsules, the other brand was $3.00 for 120 capsules. Yet, both contained the same amounts of the same active ingredients. Think about that when buying drugs. Read their labels.

A further complication in naming drugs results from the chemical similarity of many of them. A large group of drugs with different names may all really act in the same way. Nembutal is one of the over two thousand kinds of barbiturate sleeping pills that vary from one another by only a small degree in their actions on the body. Although there are some differences in the way the various barbiturates act, in terms of dosage and time of action, for the most part, they are all very similar in the nature of their actions. Each one of these different derivatives of barbituric acid will have only one generic name and at least one trade name. Quite often it will have many different trade names. Sometimes it will be known by one or more street names. The Appendix lists generic drug names with some of their proprietary names.

Another element of confusion is introduced into naming drugs because they are seldom compounded alone in commercial preparations. The vast majority of the drugs you bought in the drugstore or supermarket and a great many of those prescribed by physicians, indeed even some of those obtained illegally on the street, are not a single drug, but mixtures — two, three, four, or up to ten different drugs, in one pill or capsule. Of course we know about this from television advertising. We are often told by a very serious announcer that such-and-such a drug is a careful compounding of the ingredients most often prescribed by doctors, or again, that this particular pill has not one or two, but three, of the leading ingredients for some particular disorder. Usually, the effects of these combination products are a simple addition of the properties of each of the individual drugs that comprise the mixture. However, this is not always the case. In some circumstances, taking more than one drug at a time can either block or stop some of the properties of each drug, or in other cases, can cause them to add up to become more potent than any of the individual drugs alone. This last situation is called "potentiation" by pharmacologists. These interactions between various drugs complicate the picture of figuring out what we are taking and how much we should take.

So you can see there is great confusion surrounding the discussion of drugs. Most people don't realize that they take drugs every day. They would rather forget about it. They call what they take a "medicine," "tonic," or "beverage." Most people are uninformed about drugs. Although we take them and spend a great deal of money on them, we don't know what a drug is, don't know how it works, and probably, quite often, don't even know why we are taking it. However, to soften this rather harsh indictment, it seems only fair to point out that, if there has not been a deliberate campaign to keep us ignorant, certainly no one has taken the time, with all the claims of "drug education," to truly explain what a drug is and how it acts.

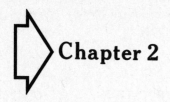

Chapter 2

Basic Principles of Drug Action

▶▶▶ WHAT YOU MUST KNOW ABOUT DRUGS

In order to take any drug with intelligence, you must know, as a rock bottom minimum, at least five major pieces of information about the drug and yourself. These are: (1) what exactly the drug is that you are about to take; (2) how much of the drug you should take, how often you should take it, and for how long a period you should continue to take it; (3) how the drug will, at the dose and on the administration schedule that you take it, affect your body, either for good or ill; (4) what signs you should watch for to know the type of effect, good or bad, you're getting from the drug; and finally, (5) while you are taking the drug, what your life situation will be; that is, what you expect to be doing and how the actions of the drug will interact with your own particular life-style. These five essential pieces of information are necessary to know before you use any drug, whether it is the early morning cup of coffee, an aspirin tablet for a headache, or a strong antibiotic that has been prescribed. Before you can ever take a drug with any safety, you must have obtained this information.

▶▶▶ WHERE TO GET DRUG INFORMATION

This raises the question as to where you can obtain valid information about drugs. Obviously, one of the first sources that you would think of is your physician. Indeed, your physician is often a very good source of information, *if you ask him.* Have him tell you what the expected effects of the drug are and how it acts. Think of taking a drug in the same way that you would think about surgery. Certainly, you would not consider having surgery performed on your body without having had an explanation of the nature of the disorder that required the surgery, a description of the surgical procedure to be performed, and what you could expect as a possible outcome of the surgery, both good and bad. A drug can cause as profound an influence on your body as surgery. You certainly should exercise the same care and demand the same kind of explanation so that you can decide whether you wish to take the drug and so that you can take the drug with intelligence and knowledge.

Another source of information is your pharmacist. Quite often, a pharmacist, though he does not diagnose illness or prescribe medications, will be a wellspring of information about the usual actions of various drugs and alternate compounds or formulations that are available. He is your primary source of information about those drugs that are obtained without a prescription. Finally, you can read books and articles on the subject of drugs. A list of good books on the subject can be found in the list of Readings.

The one piece of advice that I would certainly always follow is that, in obtaining information about drugs, as in obtaining valid information about anything else, you must consider the sources of the information. What are their motives and what do they want you to believe? For example, I don't think that you would accept the information you receive from a salesman who is trying to sell you a product with quite the same enthusiasm and confidence that you might feel from a more independent source of information with less to gain from the outcome of the dealing. Advertisers of drugs can hardly be objective. In the same way, if somebody is strongly against drugs and their use, this must be taken into consideration. Unfortunately, some people in our society do reap a profit by putting out false or misleading information about drugs.

The most common source of information about drugs for most people is their friends. This, at first blush, seems sort of ridiculous. However, it's true. Many people both receive drugs from their friends and take their advice as to how much to take or what drug to use. Since your friends know as little or less about drugs than you do, it's apparent that the information you get may not be very accurate. You may trust the motives of your friends but it's wise to question their knowledge. A friend may say to you, "Why, yes, I've had a similar condition and I took this pill that the doctor gave me. It was just right for me." But does your friend know the exact disorder for which he was being treated, whether he is competent to diagnose your disorder, whether the particular dose, or even the drug itself, is the right drug for you? Regardless of your friend's good intent, he isn't trained. This is true whether you happen to be a middle-aged suburbanite receiving the drug from your neighbor just across the way, or a more youthful drug user who obtains a pill from a friend on the street. A study performed in a suburban area near one of our major cities found that approximately one-third of the tranquilizing drugs that were taken by the residents of the community were not obtained from a physician. They were obtained from a friend who gave them a few pills and told them that this pill would make them feel better.

Whenever you take a drug you can possibly confer either benefit or harm upon yourself. Therefore, it's up to you to evaluate the potential benefit and the potential risk. You never take a drug without the expectation of benefit, but there is also always a potential for harm, however small, even with the commonest of drugs. It seems wise, then, to give at least the same thought and care to your body that you would expend if you were buying a used car. I've often heard that when you buy a used car, it is best not only to listen to what the salesman says, but also, if you're wise, to obtain an independent judgment from a professional mechanic who has both knowledge and no vital interest in selling the car. You go to this outside mechanic for precisely this reason. You want professional, expert opinion about the nature of the car you're buying so that you can consider whether it will give better service than another type, what the potential hazards are, for example, does it use too much gas, is it breakdown prone. At the same time, you want a source of information that you know you can trust because he is not trying to sell you anything. He is giving you as independent and objective a judgment as possible. In my own opinion, when you're taking a drug you ought to exhibit at least the same care by getting expert, unbiased information.

▶▶▶ **WHAT YOU MUST KNOW ABOUT THE DRUG ITSELF**

When first obtaining a drug, you will probably not know exactly what drug it is because it will be given to you under a trade name, and particularly if it was obtained by a prescription, you may not know the trade name. On the whole, knowing the trade name of the drug is not of much use since the same drug may have a hundred different trade names. Therefore, you must first find out the generic name of the drug, or, in the case of drug mixtures, the generic names of the various drugs in the mixture. The easiest way to obtain this information is by asking your physician, your pharmacist, or, in the case of drugs that you purchase without a prescription, by looking at the ingredients label on the package. Knowing the generic name lets you know what you have.

Another consideration is the vehicle and form in which the drug is given. There are a number of types of vehicles, that is, substances having no effects of their own, in which the active drug is carried. The vehicle used depends on whether the drug is to be taken by mouth, applied to the skin, injected, sniffed, dissolved under the tongue, or given through the rectum. The particular form of the drug, whether it is in solution, in a capsule or tablet, or in a dissolvable suppository, is also determined by the way it is to be administered. The following examples will help you identify particular vehicles, forms, and routes of administration.

"Tincture" or "elixir" means that the drug is carried in an alcohol solution. Examples would be "tincture of brown opium," which is known by the generic name of paregoric, or elixir terpin hydrate with codeine, which is used for coughs. Paregoric is opium dissolved in alcohol with flavoring added to make it a little more palatable. Elixir terpin hydrate is codeine dissolved in alcohol with an orange-flavored terpin hydrate syrup added to make it more palatable, to help ease tickling in the throat and to make phlegm more fluid so it is easier to cough up.

The terms "powder," "pill," or "capsule" convey only that the drugs are to be taken orally either as a loose powder, compressed into a pill, or contained in a gelatin capsule. In these cases, generally, the active drugs themselves constitute a very small part of the total powder. They are carried in a powdery vehicle such as milk sugar, which is relatively inert or innocuous to the body. Examples are aspirin "pills," sleeping powder "capsules," or antacid, dissolvable "powders." "Spansule" is one of the newer terms in the field. This indicates the drug is placed in "tiny time pills." The powder, which is the carrier and the active form of the drug, is encapsulated in a large number of very small pills that will dissolve at different rates in your stomach. Then these very small pills that are to dissolve at different rates are placed in a larger capsule. The advantage to this form of administration is that it provides a steadier and more prolonged input and action of the drug, if the dissolving rate of the pills in your stomach goes according to the way the manufacturer would like. Unfortunately, this is not always the way it ends up. There is too much variability in rates of dissolving and rates of absorption to be very sure of the precise rate at which the drug will get into your system.

Injected Drugs

The terms *intravenous, intramuscular,* and *subcutaneous* apply to drugs that are to be given in a solution by injection with a hypodermic needle. Subcutaneous refers to the injection of a drug solution just under your skin. This is the way you might receive a flu shot or a shot of morphine for pain reduction. This injection route is known by the street term "joy popping." Intramuscular injection places the drug farther into the body, into one of your deep muscles. The drug is often in an oily vehicle. In this way, it is more slowly absorbed into your bloodstream than if the same drug had been given subcutaneously. This administration technique is used when you want a longer action of the drug with a slower time of onset. It is the injection equivalent of a spansule. An example of the type of drug that might be commonly given this way is penicillin. In my own experience, these shots are quite often unpleasant and painful. The third type, intravenous injection, is not very common. It is called "mainlining" of drugs on the street. Other than this "street use," intravenous administration is usually performed in a physician's office or hospital. This is the fastest way to get a drug into the body. It goes right into the bloodstream and is quickly distributed throughout the entire body.

A problem common to all methods of giving drugs by needle is sterilization. It is very easy to cause diseases, such as serum hepatitis, if the needle has not been adequately sterilized. To overcome this problem physicians and also diabetics will often use a cheap, disposable plastic syringe which comes presterilized. Sterilization of a needle and syringe can be accomplished by soaking them for at least twenty to thirty minutes in a solution of 70 percent alcohol and water. Unfortunately, the virus that causes serum hepatitis is not killed by this method. You have to boil the needle and syringe for ten to twenty minutes to kill the serum hepatitis virus and all other germs. Then you must be very careful to extract the needle from the boiling water and place it onto the sterile syringe with a pair of sterile forceps, so that the point and shaft of the needle touch nothing and the inside of the syringe stays clean.

Topical Application of Drugs

Some drugs are applied topically. They are placed directly on the tissues to be affected. For example, ointments, lotions, sprays, oils, soaps, antiseptics, dyes, suppositories, cosmetics, nosedrops, eye-drops, eardrops, gargles, lozenges, are all directly applied. In these cases the vehicle will usually be an oil, grease, lanolin, water, or alcohol. This route of application is of limited use unless you can get the drug directly onto the tissue that you want affected. A problem can arise since some drugs that you wish to apply just to the skin are absorbed into the body through the skin. Arsenic-based cosmetics were common at one time but more recently have been outlawed because of arsenic being absorbed through the skin. The cosmetic use of arsenic caused death in some cases.

Suppositories are used to put drugs above the rectum and into the lower bowel. From here they are easily absorbed through the mucous membrane of the bowel into the bloodstream. In some cases, suppositories are used to get the drug directly to the rectal area as a topical agent. Drugs will sometimes be placed in supposi-tory form for infants who can't or won't swallow pills or liquid medicine. This is also a convenient route of administration when people are vomiting or have upset stomachs, since the drug can get into the body without being vomited back up and will not interfere with digestion. It is also a common route of drug administration for animals, eliminating the problem of getting the pill down and the pet gagging it back up.

Dissolving a pill under the tongue (sublingual) or inhaling the drug into the throat and lungs is another way to get its rapid absorption through mucous membranes, which allow chemicals to pass into the bloodstream more readily than through the skin or through the gastrointestinal tract.

Drug Age and Purity

After determining the generic ingredients in the drug you have, informing yourself as to the vehicle and the route of administration, the next thing that you must know about the drug is its purity, and in some cases, its age. The purity of a drug is determined by standards set by the Federal Food and Drug Administration (FDA). So, for the most part, you may be sure that if you obtain a drug in a drugstore or supermarket, or if it's given to you by a pharmacist, it will be free, to a reasonable degree, of any extraneous impurities. Purity standards also usually exist, but sometimes are not well enforced, for drugs taken in beverage form and for preservatives in foods. If the words USP (United States Pharmacopeia), NF (National Formulary), or NND (New and Nonofficial Drugs) are on a bottle of drugs, you may be assured that the drug has been studied and that adequate standards for its manufacture and purity have been met. Other drugs may not have these letters on them. However, that does not mean that they are impure but only that they are too new to have standards of purity published in one of the three official sources mentioned. There is no way of determining the purity of drugs received from illegal sources. This is a dangerous situation. The quality control in the clandestine laboratories that make illegal drugs is notoriously bad. There may be anything in these drugs from dirt to bird droppings, from chalk to strange, unknown poisonous materials. God knows what you receive in a drug when you have no idea of its source, purity, or conditions of manufacture.

Related to the question of the purity of a drug is its age. The length of time that a drug will be in a relatively pure and effective state depends on the nature of the coating of the pill or the kind of bottle in which it is kept, the temperature at which it has been stored, whether it has been exposed to air and other environmental factors. Sometimes changes that occur in a drug when it ages are not critical. They merely make it less potent. For example, after you have opened a bottle of aspirin, moisture gets into it from the air. This moisture combines with the aspirin (which is usually a compressed powder) to produce compounds which have neither beneficial nor harmful effects. Therefore, if a bottle of aspirin has been around for a long period of time after it has been opened, the pills in it won't harm you, but they may not do you much good, either, because of a loss of potency. If a tablet is coated with a hard cover, or if it's in a capsule, it generally lasts longer.

Sometimes the age of a drug is very important since it not only may lose its potency but also may become dangerous due to chemical changes. If this is the case, a label showing the expiration date will be on every bottle of such a drug. This is important to look for because you don't want to take a drug that has passed its expiration date. An example of problems associated with old drugs that happened recently is an outbreak of liver disorders, particularly in the families of physicians. When the situation was investigated it was shown that the physicians had been given samples of an antibiotic. They had kept these samples in their desks or in their homes for quite a period of time, past the date the drugs had expired, and had then given these old antibiotics to members of their own families. In this particular case, when the drug became aged, it was a dangerous liver poison. This is just an illustration of what can happen if you use a drug that is over age. It also shows that physicians are human and can make careless mistakes just like everybody else.

The effect that you get from a drug depends not only on its type but also on the amount of the drug that you take, how often you take it, and for how long a period you take it. That the amount of drug you take is important is well known. Everybody knows that it is impossible for an adult to become drunk on three drops of whiskey. On the other hand, anybody would be drunk if he drank eight ounces of pure alcohol all at one time. This illustrates how different the effect of a drug can be, depending on how much is taken. Often when people discuss drugs, they will describe in detail what a drug does without ever mentioning how much of the drug is taken. This failure to specify the dose of drug generates a great deal of confusion. You can't intelligently discuss the benefits of a drug or the dangers of a drug without specifying dose. You can take too much of anything. You can be killed if you drink too much water at one time. Indeed, that fact was the basis of one of the old torture techniques. Yet, the right amount of water is necessary for the maintenance of life. So, drug dose is something that is always of concern in talking about drugs or considering the use of drugs for yourself. How much of the drug gives what kind of an effect?

In discussing the relation between the amount given and the effect produced, pharmacologists refer to the "dose-response" curve. This curve is plotted as illustrated in Figure 1. Dose is usually specified in milligrams or milliliters (mg or ml). (See Table 1 for abbreviations and weight and measure equivalents.) The upright axis shows the degree of effect of the drug and the horizontal axis indicates the amount of drug that yields that effect. The curve for almost any drug follows the lazy-S pattern shown. If a drug is less potent, the entire curve will be shifted to the right. If a drug is more potent it will shift the curve to the left. You might think of this in the same way you would consider beer, wine, and whiskey. Whiskey is a more potent drug than beer. That is to say, it takes a

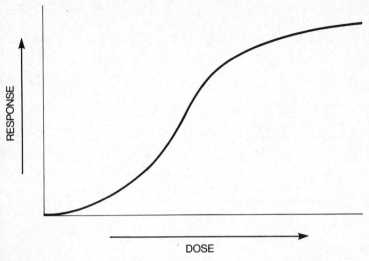

▶ FIGURE 1

Dose-Response Curve
The ordinate represents an increase in the body's response to the drug. The abscissa represents increasing dose of the drug. The S-curve is the effect of increasing dose on bodily response.

smaller amount, or dose, of whiskey to produce a particular level of intoxication than does beer.

Wine is in between whiskey and beer in potency. The dose-response curves in Figure 2 show this relationship. Wine is in the middle, beer has a curve shifted to the right, and whiskey a curve shifted to the left. It doesn't change the effect of the drug to be more or less potent, it just changes the amount necessary to be taken to achieve a particular degree of effect. A drug is not necessarily better, more dangerous, or anything else just because it is more potent than another drug. It merely means that it takes a smaller amount of the drug to get an effect than it would of a less potent one.

There are three characteristics of the S-shaped, dose-response curve that are important to consider. First, there is the bottom, flat

▶ TABLE 1

Abbreviations, Weights, Measures, and Equivalents

Abbreviations

kg	kilogram
gm	gram
mg	milligram
mcg	microgram
ml	milliliter
l	liter
oz	ounce
lb	pound
ppm	parts per million

Weights and Equivalents (Approximate)

100 mcg equals about three granules of fine sugar
1 mcg equals 1/1,000,000 of a gram
1 mg equals 1,000 mcg
1 gm equals 1,000 mg or 1/32 ounce
1 kg equals 1,000 gm or 2.2 lbs.
1 grain (Apothecary) equals 65 mg
1 ounce equals 480 grains or about 28,800 mg

Measures and Equivalents (Approximate)

1 ounce equals 30 ml
1 teaspoon equals 8 ml
1 tablespoon equals 15 ml
1 liter equals 1,000 ml

EXAMPLE: A standard 5-grain-aspirin tablet equals about 300 mg of aspirin or about 3/32 of an ounce of active drug.

portion of the S where increases in dose don't yield any increase in response. In fact, doses at these levels produce no response at all. These are called "subthreshold" doses. This shows that you must take a certain amount of drug before you start getting an effect. Just

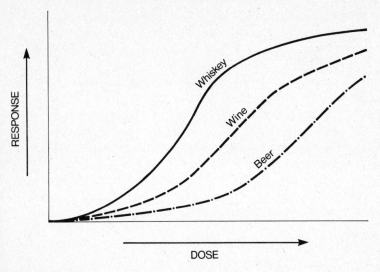

▶ FIGURE 2

Dose-Response Curves for Drugs of Different Potencies
The ordinate represents an increase in the body's response to the drugs. The abscissa represents increasing dose of the drugs.

about at the bottom part of the S, where the curve accelerates very rapidly, a dose of the drug starts to produce an important degree of effect. This point is called the "threshold" dose. The threshold dose shows how much drug you must take to get any effect at all. After this point, the increase in response is in proportion to the amount of drug taken.

The next part of the curve is its almost linear portion going up toward the top. This portion of the curve indicates how much more drug you must take to get any desired increase in the amount of effect. The flatter the S-curve the more drug must be taken to get an increase in effect. The more vertical the curve, the more the effect will go up with even a small additional dose of drug. This part of the curve shows how carefully you must monitor the dose you take. If you have a drug that has a rather flat curve it means that you can vary the dose a great deal with only a small degree of change in the amount of effect you get. Thus, you can be less careful with your dose. On the other hand, if you have a drug that has an S that is almost straight up and down, even a very small change in dose can tremendously change the effect you get. Obviously, then, you must be much more careful in getting the dose just right. Logically, more potent drugs usually have more vertical dose-response curves.

The upper part of the S-curve flattens again. This shows that there is some dose of drug at which, even though you take more drug, you're not going to get any more effect of the kind that you desire. This is called the "ceiling dose" of the drug. If you take a drug at doses beyond its ceiling dose it does absolutely no good in terms of the effect that you're trying to obtain. Indeed, taking more might cause problems. There are always other effects of a drug besides those wanted. These other effects could have very differently shaped dose-response curves. As an example, studies have shown that aspirin has a threshold dose of about 200 mg and a ceiling dose at an amount of about 900 mg for adults for relief of simple pain. Nine hundred mg is about the equivalent of three standard aspirin tablets. So for the normal use of the aspirin, such as headache relief, it doesn't do any good to ever take more than three aspirin at one time. If you take more than three aspirin, you may produce effects that you do not want and you will not increase the amount of pain relief that is obtained. (I should add, as a cautionary note, that for relief in true arthritis there is a different dose-response curve than there is for simple pain relief for aspirin.) Another effect of aspirin is to cause ringing noises in the ears. The threshold dose for this effect is about 4 gm per day. For obvious reasons, no one has tried to determine the ceiling dose for this particular effect.

All drugs have more than one effect. You usually take a drug for only one of the various things that it does to your body. Further, different effects of the same drug can have different dose-response curves. The curves can differ in their position on the graph, that is, potency, and they can differ in the shape or slope of the curve.

When considering all the different actions of a drug you must include those that you don't want as well as those you want. You must try to find that dose which will give you the effect wanted without producing too much of any of the effects that are not wanted. To do this, you have to know approximately where you are on each of the dose-response curves for each of the effects. As an example, I enjoy drinking Scotch. I have found that approximately two ounces of Scotch are relaxing and set up my appetite for dinner. On the other hand, there is an effect of whiskey that I don't want. I have determined that with a dose of about five ounces of Scotch I will wake up, either in the middle of the night or in the morning, feeling queasy and exhausted. Therefore, I always have to take this into account when drinking — knowing that the dose of 2 ounces of Scotch produces the effects I want but the dose of 5 ounces of Scotch produces a lot of effects I don't want. I have a margin of error of 3 ounces in between.

Time to Onset and Length of Drug Action

Another consideration related to dose is the time-action curve of a drug for a particular effect. It takes some amount of time after you have taken a drug before it will reach its peak effect. It then stays at a plateau level for a while and, finally, slowly starts to decline in its action until the effect has gone. The time-action curves of drugs are influenced by a number of factors: first, the amount of the drug taken; second, the manner in which it is taken; third, the rate at which the drug is destroyed in the body; fourth, the condition of the body when the drug is taken. For example, if you take a drink of alcohol on an empty stomach, you know that you can feel its effects much more rapidly than if you take it on a full stomach. Food in your stomach slows the absorption of the drug alcohol. The same is true for almost any other drug that you take orally. If your stomach is full, the absorption rate of the drug will be a good deal slower. For example, a full stomach slows the absorption of barbiturate

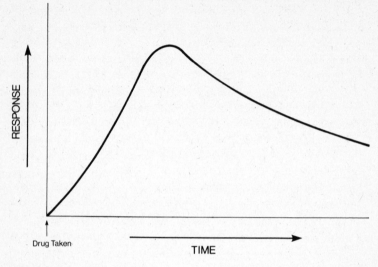

▶ FIGURE 3

Time-Action Curve
The ordinate represents an increase in the body's response to the drug. The abscissa represents the passage of time. The time-action curve depicts the effect of time on the body's response to the drug.

sleeping pills to six times the length it takes on an empty stomach. For the most part, you can expect any solid drug that you take by the oral route on an empty stomach to take between fifteen and forty-five minutes to reach its peak effect.

The form of the drug can also influence its rate of absorption from the stomach. For example, if you take aspirin in a carbonated form, as with some of the commercial preparations that bubble, or if you dissolve regular aspirin in hot water, the drug will reach its peak concentration in the blood in about ten to fifteen minutes. If the drug is taken as a compressed pill rather than in a liquid form, it may take about fifteen to forty-five minutes. However, in considering these various forms of the drug you might use you should remember that the condition of your stomach, such as whether you've had food recently, is far more important for absorption time than the particular form in which you take the drug.

The fastest means of getting a drug into the system is by intravenous injection. When it is necessary to have drug effects within seconds the drug will be certain to get into the body rapidly when put directly into the bloodstream. On the other hand, the time-action of an intravenous administration is usually short. An intramuscular injection is used when slow absorption and long lasting-time are wanted of a drug that is not absorbed easily through the stomach and therefore can't be taken orally. Many drugs either cannot be absorbed through the stomach at all or, at least, are very badly absorbed by that route. In this case, the drug is usually carried in an oily vehicle. It is injected deeply into the muscle. From here the drug will slowly diffuse out of the muscle into the bloodstream over a considerable period of hours. This extends the time-action of the drug as well as slowing its onset time. As a general rule of thumb you may say that the faster a drug takes effect, the faster it will be eliminated from your body, and the more slowly the onset, the more slowly a drug is eliminated from your body.

Sometimes you want to have both a long time-action and a rapid onset, for example, with an antibiotic. To achieve this a drug may be given simultaneously by two different routes. It is not uncommon to have a shot of penicillin just under the skin (subcutaneously), which is a relatively fast onset route, and also take a pill, an orally absorbable form of penicillin, or an intramuscular injection of penicillin to ensure a longer time-action.

The downward slope of the time-action curve indicates that all drugs are eliminated from the body. There are many different means by which the body eliminates drugs. They range from very active processes in which the body grabs the drug molecules, detoxifies them by changing them chemically, and ships them out as quickly as it can. There are also slower methods used by the body. With these slower methods it usually takes about seventy-two hours for the drug to slowly diffuse away from the body tissues. Whether there are active bodily agents to eliminate a drug sometimes depends on the particular condition of your body. For example, if you've taken a drug for quite a while, you may have developed a condition of "tolerance" to the drug. This often means that taking the drug has caused your body to form specific antagonistic chemicals (enzymes) that help you detoxify and eliminate the drug. A person who has developed tolerance will require more drug more often to get the same degree of effect as before he became tolerant, that is, the dose-response curve is shifted to the right. Another point to note is that the liver is the major site for the detoxification of drugs within your body before they are eliminated. If you have any of the liver disorders, such as jaundice or hepatitis, so that your liver is not functioning correctly, drug time-action can be vastly changed. In this case, when you take a drug it may not be detoxified and it may be eliminated from your body very slowly. In this situation it's very easy to get an overdose because the drug has little downward portion to the time-action curve. A second dose of the drug just doubles the problem. This is one of the reasons that when you are seriously ill a physician will often do liver function tests. It is not that he is worried about your liver causing the disease, but he wants to make sure that your liver is functioning well, so that any drug that is given to you can be detoxified and eliminated in the expected manner.

In advertising, a great deal of importance is attached to the onset time and time-action of drugs. There are many assertions that one pain reliever gets to the source of a headache much faster than another. Usually, there is some basis in fact for these claims. In the case of a buffered aspirin, the buffering compound causes the pill to disintegrate more rapidly in your stomach. Therefore, it shortens absorption to about ten minutes compared to about twenty minutes for plain aspirin tablets. On the other hand, if you take the aspirin in a liquid form, either as a carbonated, bubbling form or in hot water, you will have the same rapid absorption. Anyway, the condition of fullness of your stomach is more important as a factor in absorption time. Many people expect too quick an effect from an oral drug. Also, they sometimes expect a drug to work for a longer period of time than it can. Let's again take the example of aspirin. If you take three aspirin tablets you have taken its ceiling dose for simple pain reduction. It won't do you any good to take any more than this. It just won't help. You must expect to wait up to forty-five minutes for the peak action if you take it in a simple, compressed tablet form and if you have food in your stomach. Aspirin has a time-action of four to six hours. The range is wide because different people can eliminate aspirin at different rates. But you can expect at least three good hours of a fairly strong level of pain reduction. There is no use, no need, and indeed, potential harm in taking more aspirin before the three to four hours are up. Even after three hours, if you take more aspirin, you're probably still on the descending limb of the time-action curve of your first dose so that in another forty-five minutes, as the first dose curve is beginning to get low, you have reinstigated a full level of pain reduction again. Figure 4 shows a graphic analysis of this time-action.

As another example of a time-action curve, let us consider alcohol. The average person, with an empty stomach, will begin to get an effect from alcohol in about ten to fifteen minutes. The peak effects occur in approximately forty-five minutes. Alcohol is detoxified at the rate of about 1 ounce per hour. You can see that if you drink at a rate of approximately 1 ounce per hour you will achieve a constant level of about ½ to ¾ ounce in your body at any one time. You will never truly become drunk because your body is detoxifying the drug at about the same rate you're taking it in. You'll get a little peak as it comes up to its full concentration, but it will start right down again. On the other hand, if you drink alcohol at a rate faster than 1 ounce an hour, then you can expect to start to get drunk because alcohol accumulates in your body faster than it can eliminate the drug. The time-action curves in Figure 5 illustrate these points. The rate at which you consume the drug can govern the effect that you get from it — not only how much you take, but also how fast you take it.

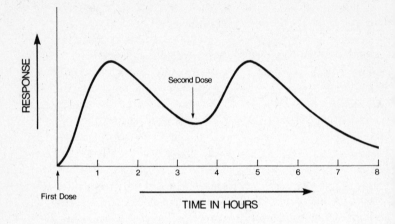

Time-Action of Two Doses of a Drug
The ordinate represents an increase in the body's response to the drug. The abscissa represents the passage of time. The time-action curve depicts the effect of time on the body's response to two doses of a drug.

Schedule of Administration

The third consideration in relation to drug dose and time-action is the schedule of administration. You rarely take only one dose of a drug. The schedule of administration is how often you take the drug and how long you keep taking it, that is, the total number of doses that you take. Here I'm not only referring to the amount you take in a few hours as with alcohol, but use of the drug over days, weeks, or months. The schedule of administration governs the amount of drug accumulated in your body and the total time of effective action.

In many cases, to achieve the desired effect, it is necessary to maintain an adequate level of the drug in your bloodstream for a

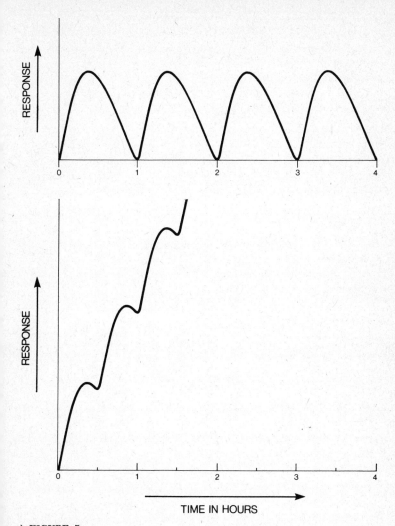

Time-Action of Multiple Drug Doses
The ordinates represent an increase in the body's response to the drug. The abscissas represent the passage of time. The time-action curves depict the noncumulative and the cumulative effects of multiple doses of a drug.

prolonged period. Colonies of germs are not destroyed totally by a single dose of antibiotic. Pain from an injury is not eliminated until the injury is repaired. Most malfunctions of your body cannot be corrected in the few hours that the single dose of a drug may last. Even if you feel better immediately after taking a drug, it is no reason to cease medication. Some people think they are being noble by cutting their drug dose from the one prescribed. Some even think they are acting wisely when they cease taking their drug, without consulting their physicians. Most of the time, they are making a very serious mistake. Even if they feel better the problem may still be there.

Drug Tolerance

A factor in a drug administration schedule is the development of tolerance. Tolerance to a drug occurs when it requires a higher dose to get the same degree of response as previously, that is, a right shift in the dose-response curve. You can become tolerant to many drugs if you take them repeatedly. Sometimes, this is due to the development of specific antagonist chemicals (enzymes) to the drug that detoxify it so it is more rapidly eliminated from the body. It may also be that the body cells the drug acts upon become less sensitive to it with repeated exposure. The individual cells of your body can adjust to drugs. Tolerance causes no qualitative change in the drug's effect, it just takes more drug to get it. Tolerance is generally not too great a problem. You can always take a bit more drug to get the effect you want. On the other hand, the rate at which tolerance develops for the desired effects of a drug is often different from the rate at which tolerance develops to undesired drug effects. If the desired effects are rapidly tolerated and the adverse effects slowly tolerated, you have a problem. Soon the possibility of undesirable effects will outweigh the advantages of the drug at the required dose. The margin of error between a lethal dose of a drug and its effective dose can become quite small. Sleeping pills are a good illustration of this point. You may become tolerant to their effects in causing sleep, but tolerance to their lethal effects develops at a much slower rate. So, your margin of safety becomes quite small. This margin of safety is called the "therapeutic safety ratio." It is a comparison of the dose of drug that will yield the effect you want to the dose that's necessary to kill you. It is usually stated as a ratio. For example, the therapeutic safety ratio for a barbiturate sleeping pill in a nontolerant person is about 1:10. It takes ten times as much to kill you as it does to produce sleep. But if you become tolerant to the drug, the therapeutic safety ratio changes so that it becomes about one in two, that is, it will take two times as much to kill you as to achieve the effect you desire. As you can see, when the therapeutic safety ratio becomes smaller your chances of getting the effect you want, and not death, become less certain.

Drug Dependence

Another factor that is associated with the administration schedule of a drug is "dependence." Dependence on drugs is a confusing topic because many people *think* they know about it. In its most general sense, dependence is defined as the desire of a person to continue to take a drug of any kind for some expected benefit. Often dependence is broken down into two types. "Psychological dependence," or "habit," means that the person won't have any drastic physiological upset if he doesn't take the drug, but that he does want to take it and will seek the drug because he expects some type of benefit. Psychological dependence exists for almost all of the drugs that will relieve pain. It exists for drugs that make a person feel better. One of the worst, strongest, and most prevalent psychological dependences in this country is on laxatives. Also, for a large number of people, organic foods, vitamins, minerals, and many other drugs are habitually taken with the belief that they confer benefit. These are psychological dependences.

The other type of dependence is called "physical dependence." If you've taken some drugs for an adequate period of time, at a high enough dose, often enough, your body changes in such a way that if you cease to take the drug there will be some degree of physiological upset. Perhaps one of the mildest forms of physical dependence is on the caffeine in coffee, tea, cocoa, or cola drinks. A relatively large number of people have formed a physical dependence upon coffee to the extent that if they cease to take it they will get a headache. This is due to the changes in the cells of their brain. They actually come to require coffee. The headache is not a severe disorder and it will go away in a few days. Most people can tolerate a headache for a while, but it is an example of true physical dependence on a drug. The nicotine in cigarettes also produces physical dependence. It has been shown that there are changes in brain waves when you cease smoking after you've smoked for years. These, of course, also go away after a little while with no apparent problems. It's not that the physiological changes are permanent. Very few of the physiological upsets associated with physical dependence last very long. The name for these upsets that occur upon the cessation of taking a drug that produces physical dependence is "the withdrawal syndrome."

Alcohol and barbiturates, either singly or acting together, cause a physical dependence if taken in an adequate quantity, often enough, over a period of months or years. The withdrawal syndrome can be very severe. If the alcohol or barbiturate sleeping pills are withdrawn suddenly, after long and heavy use, death results in about 15 percent of those cases not under medical care. Also, the potent drugs for the reduction of pain, the opiates, cause physical dependence if taken in a high enough dose, often enough, for at least ten days. Usually, dependence on opiates is developed over a period of weeks or months. There is not as severe a physiological upset upon abrupt withdrawal of an opiate as with barbiturates or alcohol. It can cause about 1 to 3 percent deaths in severely dependent, ill people if not conducted under medical care. Cessation of opiate taking causes about seventy-two hours of very unpleasant sensations. Withdrawal does not involve running around and screaming, as it is often seen in movies. The person during withdrawal lies on the bed, bent double, groaning with stomach cramps, sweating, and dilated pupils.

In this discussion of dependence I have not used the term "addiction." There is a reason for this. In 1965, the World Health Organization decided that the term "addiction" meant so many different things to different people that it was almost meaningless. Therefore, for an accurate description of drug actions you should not use the term "addiction," but rather use the term "dependence." Then the type of dependence must be defined specifically, in relation to the drug and the life pattern of the person who chronically takes that drug. Certainly, the term "addiction" names one of the areas in which a great deal more heat than light has been generated by many of the so-called "drug-education" programs and the self-appointed drug experts of our society.

▶▶▶ INDIVIDUAL FACTORS AFFECTING DRUG ACTIONS

One major factor that has to be considered when discussing drugs is the individual response of each person to any given drug at a particular dose, on a particular schedule of administration. Each of us is somewhat unique in reference to physiology, chemistry, and life-style. Therefore, since a drug always acts in combination with a specific physiology and life pattern, there are going to be some individual differences in drug effects. Further, the same person differs in physiology, chemistry, and life-style under different circumstances, for example, when there is disease or fatigue, or when driving a car, and so on. So you can't expect the action from a particular dose of a specific drug to be exactly the same twice in a row. It will be similar but not exactly the same.

Drug Dose and Body Size

There are certain things about you that are known to markedly influence drug action. For example, how big you are. Most drugs, after entering the bloodstream, are distributed throughout the entire body. The drug goes to your big toe, to your lung, to your brain, and the rest of you fairly evenly. The drug is not going to be active at all spots of the body. Indeed, there will be only a few target sites at which the drug will be active. Because of this, the bigger you are, as a given dose of a drug is distributed through your body, the less drug will get to the specific target sites at which it has its major activity. In calculating drug dose to achieve a given effect, the size of the individual has to be taken into account. Often this is expressed as milligrams of the drug to the number of kilograms of weight of the person. Ordinarily, for the adult male, body weight is estimated at an average of 70 kg, that is, 2.2 kg per pound or 154 pounds. The drug dose is calculated on that basis. However, if a person is small, perhaps weighs only 50 kg, the drug dose would have to be reduced appropriately to achieve the same effect that a larger dose would have in a 70-kg person.

Drug Dose and Age

Another factor that is taken into account individually is the age of the person receiving the drug. Generally, far less drug is needed for a person below twelve years of age or above sixty-five years of age. Indeed, some drugs are particularly potent in infants and young children. The dose must be adjusted very carefully. A young child, or an infant, is both a very small person and a person whose chemistry has not matured. A standard formula has been worked out for the age and size factors to determine the dose of a drug to be given to a child. The easiest way to account for size is to take the usual dose prescribed for a 70-kg person and reduce it in proportion to the weight of the child. This is *not* an appropriate formula for very young children or for infants. Their nervous and other bodily systems have not yet fully developed. It is useful for children between the ages of five and twelve. After the age of twelve a child is considered an adult in terms of drug dose. A physician should figure the dose of all medicine for children below the age of five. There are just too many possible complicating factors involved.

Drug Dose and Sex

Another factor that enters into the action of some drugs is sex. First, women tend to be smaller than males, though obviously this is not always true. A special situation comes about because of the female menstrual cycle. At certain times of the month there are higher levels of the female hormones in the body. These can interact with some drugs. Also, many females tend to be borderline anemics while they are menstruating, due to blood loss. Finally, special problems can occur when taking drugs during pregnancy. We've had one of our most celebrated drug cases in this area, thalidomide. Thalidomide was believed to be a safe drug for use as a sleeping compound. Many studies in Europe had shown it to have a much more favorable therapeutic safety ratio than the barbiturates. It's very difficult to kill anyone with an overdose of thalidomide. Therefore, thalidomide offered what appeared to be a number of marked advantages over barbiturate sleeping pills. Unfortunately, as was found out, if thalidomide is taken during the first three months of pregnancy, it can cause the development of abnormalities in the fetus. This is a particularly difficult problem. Many women don't know that they are pregnant during the first three months. This is an illustration of a distinctly sex-linked drug effect. Thalidomide can be a useful drug for males, since males do not get pregnant, but in the pregnant female, it causes trouble. It's too bad that thalidomide had to be completely pulled from the market, since it does offer some advantages over barbiturates as a sleeping pill. It is a drug that should not be used for a female during her childbearing years. But that, perhaps, should not have caused its prohibition for use with males or older females. I suppose it's safer the way it is now. If thalidomide were available at all, I imagine accidents would have occurred. In general, the fewer drugs taken during pregnancy the better. Many drugs may affect an unborn child. Our knowledge in this area is too skimpy for one to feel very secure about almost any drug.

Drug Dose and Physiological State

Your particular condition at a time that you take a drug can have a marked effect on the way the drug acts. For example, your diet will interact with some drugs to produce some rather unusual effects. This makes a lot of sense when you stop and think about it. Drugs work by acting on your natural bodily mechanisms. They interact with the chemistry of the body. Your chemistry partly comes from what you eat. A spectacular illustration of this kind of interaction of drugs with diet occurred in what has been called the "Italian syndrome." Some of the older types of antidepressant drugs acted by blocking the metabolism of some amino acids in the body. Amino acids are contained in most of the food you eat and are essential for your survival. Your body can manufacture some of them but others have to come from your diet. One particular amino acid, called tyramine, which has its metabolism blocked by the older anti-depressant drugs, became important in some drug poisoning cases. A number of people came into hospitals with high fever and high blood pressure. In a few cases, the people died due to excessive temperature and high blood pressure. It was noticed that most of these patients were Italian and were taking the type of antidepres-sant drug that blocked the metabolism of the amino acid tyramine. It finally was realized that some Italians have a tremendous quantity of tyramine in their diets. They eat a much higher level of it than people of other cultural backgrounds, in the form of Bel Paese cheese, Chianti wine, and fava beans. All these are loaded with tyramine. The drug blocked the metabolism of the tyramine, which caused an excessive buildup of this amino acid, resulting in high blood pressure and fever. The "Italian syndrome" really was tyramine poisoning. Thus, we can say that with the older antide-pressant drugs, now rarely used, a diet high in cheese, wine, and fava beans is contraindicated. This again illustrates that to be able to have some reasonable idea of what a drug is going to do, you have to understand your own individual situation and how the drug will interact with your condition.

A fourth type of information that should be considered: the possible unwanted reactions that can be caused by the drug. These are generally lumped under the term "adverse drug reactions." It is important for you to know what the odds are that you will have an adverse reaction to a drug. Whenever you take a drug, you are presumably seeking some benefit. You are also taking the risk of adverse reactions. There is no drug that does not have some degree of risk associated with its use. There is no drug, or drug use pattern, that can be regarded as totally safe. It's only a matter of degree of risk of undesired adverse reactions. Many times it will be up to you to judge the potential benefit that you expect from a drug and to weigh this against the risk of some adverse reaction. Then you must consider how adverse the "adverse reaction" is for you. How desirable the potential benefit is.

There are many types of adverse reactions to drugs but some are common to all drugs. They are something that you should watch for whenever you take any drug. First is one called hypersensitivity. Some people are hypersensitive to some drugs. They can take a very low dose of a drug but get a large effect. The effect is of the same kind as expected, but much, much stronger than would usually be expected for the drug at that dose. In reference to the dose-response curve, then, a hypersensitive individual is one who has the usual dose-response curve shifted to the left. As an example, the usual stimulant dose of amphetamines is 5 to 10 milligrams. As it happens, I am hypersensitive to amphetamines. A dose of half that much, 2.5 milligrams, is enough to keep me active for about six hours. This shows that hypersensitivity means getting the effect that is expected but it takes a much lower dose to yield the expected effect. So, if you take the usual dose, you get much more effect than you desire.

A second type of adverse effect is called an "idiosyncratic" response, or "atypical" response. This means that you don't react the way most people do with the drug. You may even get the opposite reaction from the drug from the one usually experienced. One common illustration of this phenomenon is with sleeping pills. There are some people, particularly children, who take a sleeping pill and instead of becoming depressed, sedated, and sleepy, become stimulated and elated. A sleeping pill will cause some children to tear around the room as though they've been zapped with a bolt of electricity. Thus, the "idiosyncratic," or "atypical," response is different from the one that was expected. It is not just a shifting of the dose-response curve. This is a new and unexpected effect. This type of response is fairly common with drugs that affect the mind. It is reasonably uncommon with other kinds of drugs.

Drug Allergy (Hypersensitivity)

A third type of adverse reaction is the allergic response to a drug. An allergic response can be the most dangerous adverse reaction that can occur with a drug. It can occur with any drug. An allergic response occurs when any chemical substance, and it need not be a drug, acts upon your body in such a way that your body responds to it as if it were an infection. The mechanisms of defense of the body that are responsible for fighting infections are called into play. There is a release of the chemicals in your body, particularly histamine, that are beneficial in fighting infection. But in this case, there is no infection to fight.

The most serious form of allergic response is shock. In this adverse reaction the blood pressure falls precipitously as all the blood vessels expand. In the extreme case of this blood pressure drop, the heart cannot maintain its function. Death can occur within a couple of minutes. Luckily, this is a rather rare reaction. Very few people are so allergic to a drug that they have the full shock reaction to it. In most cases it is a lethal reaction since the person is not close enough to a medical facility to be pulled out of it.

Other forms of drug allergies are much more common. I recently went through a bout of allergy. First, I developed the classic allergy signs that are present when the body reacts to a foreign chemical by the release of histamine. I itched, and when I scratched I produced long, flaring, red streaks that didn't just go away. After I'd scratched two or three times, large wheals formed in these areas. This is the triad of histamine symptoms — itch, flare, wheal. A wheal is easy to recognize. It is large, from the size of a quarter to that of a plate. It is soft and puffy. It is red or white and it itches like hell. My reaction became severe, and it spread from a relatively small area on my arms to my entire body. At this time, I went into the hospital. There was a good reason for going into the hospital at this time, since the next allergy symptom I developed was swelling in my throat, a potentially dangerous condition. The histamine caused the blood vessels in my throat to dilate, causing the tissue in the throat to swell. This made swallowing uncomfortable and painful. In some cases, the swelling in the throat can be so severe that it presses into the windpipe, and breathing is not possible without an open wind-pipe. This swelling, when it starts to get potentially life threatening, is called "angioneurotic edema." I then developed the third major symptom of allergy, called "serum sickness." I got a steady, low-grade fever and aching joints. My body was fighting back with a fever as if I had an infection though I had no evidence of any infection whatsoever. Mine was a fairly classic allergic reaction. It would have been the pattern that would be expected for a drug, a food, or any other chemical that might be ingested to which you are quite allergic. Anything put on the skin is particularly liable to set off such a reaction. Generally, the allergic rash is small and localized, but the reaction can become severe and kill. So it's something always to watch for. If you're taking any drug and you start to develop the itch, flare, wheal triad, stop taking the drug and get professional help immediately. It can get serious.

The fifth thing you must know before taking a drug is how the drug effects will interact with your own particular life-style. This is a complex topic. Each of you has a particular life-style. When you take a drug, changes will occur in your body that may either help you do what you want or hinder you. Let me give you an example. If you have hayfever, a form of allergy, and you take antihistamine-type drugs, you expect to be able to live your life with less inconvenience, less wheezing, less stopped-up nose, and, in general, more comfortably. On the other hand, you may also wish to drive a car, operate a piece of machinery of some kind and stay awake and alert. Most antihistamines also cause sedation and drowsiness, particularly if taken in conjunction with alcohol. Therefore, you must weigh the advantages and disadvantages. If you take the drug you may do away with one set of unpleasant symptoms but cause another set. If you have to drive a car it may be dangerous to take the drug because it can interfere with your ability to drive safely.

It's up to you to weigh the benefits and the problems attendant on using the drug. You have a life that you want to live in a certain way. You take a drug with the expectation that it will benefit you in living the way you wish. You then must know about the drug itself, its effects upon you as an individual, the correct dosage, its time-action, the proper schedule of administration, and its potential adverse reactions in order to maximize the chance that the drug will be useful for you and not detrimental to you in the way that you want to live. It is the usage pattern of a drug that gives it a potential for benefit or potential for harm. There may be some usage pattern, with the right dose, the right drug, the right schedule of administration, that can give a greater chance of benefit than harm. There are always risks. You must do a benefit-risk analysis. In cooperation with your physician or your pharmacist, ask the questions that will enable you to make a wise decision. What are the possibilities? What are the odds that a particular drug, at a particular amount, on a given schedule of administration will confer benefit to you? What are the odds that the drug, in this pattern of use, might cause reactions that you do not want? It's your body, so it's up to you to find out. Nobody else is going to have to live with it.

To summarize these basic principles that apply to all drugs, you have to consider: (1) what the drug is, its purity and its form or route of administration; (2) you must know its dose-response curve for its different types of effects, time-action curves, and the effects of different schedules of administration; (3) you must understand the different individual factors in your condition, diet, other drugs you are taking, etc., that interact with the drug; (4) you must have an appreciation for potential adverse affects that are caused by the drug, and (5) you must consider how the drug actions will interact with your own desired life-style. This is the minimum information that you must have to take a drug with wisdom.

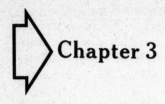

Chapter 3

Sleeping Pills

Sleep that knits up the ravell'd sleeve of care, the death of each day's life, sore labour's bath, balm of hurt minds, great nature's second course, chief nourisher in life's feast. Act II, Scene I, *Macbeth*

Thus, in his story of Macbeth, Shakespeare poignantly describes the blessings of sleep. In this description of sleep, Macbeth expresses a feeling commonly experienced by all of us at times in our lives. We, of this modern era, are not unique in this wish to be able to find relief in sleep. The Eber Papyrus, which describes medicine used in the Middle Kingdom of Egypt about 1000 B.C., mentions the use of drugs derived from the poppy plant to induce sleep in patients suffering with pain. The opium poppy's Latin name, *Papaver somniferum,* means "poppy of sleep." Also in early Egypt, alcoholic beverages were used to induce sleep. These were as commonly used by the people of that day as they are by the citizens of today to ease their minds from the weariness of daily life struggles.

Modern sleep remedies began with the discovery that salts of bromide would cause a slowing of activity in the central nervous system that induced sleep. The first preparation of bromide salt was produced in 1857. By the early 1870s, in London, tons of bromides were being produced to be used in so-called "nerve tonics." In the United States, bromides were also being used in massive amounts. At that time, the dangers of bromide poisoning were not appreciated. Lately, the use of bromides as sleep-inducing preparations has almost entirely been eliminated owing to the number of poisonings caused by these bromide drugs. We do still have drugs that use names associated with the bromides, for example, Bromo-Seltzer. However, these compounds no longer contain bromide salts.

Chloral hydrate was discovered in 1875 and, soon after that, paraldehyde, a similar drug. Since chloral hydrate is a form of chloroform, it was thought to cause sleep by changing into chloroform in the blood. This theory has since been disproven. Chloral hydrate acts by a different mechanism from chloroform, one much more closely related to alcohol's mechanism of action than to chloroform's. Finally, in 1903, barbiturates were introduced into our storehouse of sleep-producing agents. The use of barbiturates was made possible by the work of a twenty-nine-year-old research assistant who had first synthesized barbituric acid a few years before. This young research assistant was Adolph von Bayer, for whom the giant Bayer Pharmaceutical Company has been named. Although barbituric acid itself does not induce sleep, it was its discovery that allowed later investigators to be able to synthesize the over two thousand five hundred different kinds of barbiturates that have now been produced.

▶▶▶ THE NATURE OF SLEEP

It is surprising that we know so little about a phenomenon as common as sleep. We do know that individuals vary tremendously in their sleep needs. In research studies conducted in the Antarctic during the winter, when it was always dark and people lived in huts built under the ice, in a circumstance where each person could adjust his own sleep schedule to whatever pattern he desired, there were tremendous differences in the voluntary patterns of sleep of different individuals. Some people would sleep about twelve hours a day, whereas others dropped down to about five hours' sleep a day. Again, some people would sleep all in one stretch, while others would catnap, off and on, throughout the twenty-four hours. All of them, whatever pattern they happened to choose, seemed to do quite well. In some cases, they were happier with their own particular sleep cycle than when they were back in civilization where they had been on the standard eight-hour sleep pattern. This demonstrates that the need for sleep varies a tremendous amount in different people. The best possible pattern of sleep for an optimum feeling of well-being is different for different people. Other studies have confirmed this variability in the need for sleep. There certainly is nothing sacred about getting eight hours of sleep a night. It may be that you, as an individual, require more, or it may be that you require less. It may be that you will be happier sleeping all at one time or, possibly, catnaps are better for you. However, one limit seemed to have been established. It takes about four hours of sleep per twenty-four hours, as a rockbottom minimum for the maintenance of health and a feeling of well-being. Less sleep than that for anyone will cause problems. Further, we know that people who are depressed or who have a great many problems on their minds require more sleep. It seems that there is a physiological requirement by your body, just due to the sheer process of living, for at least four hours of sleep per twenty-four hours. On the other hand, if you're unhappy, worried, nervous, or upset, you may require additional sleep to help you dissipate the effects of this unhappiness or worry. We also know that most people can go without sleep for up to seventy-two hours with little or no harm. The younger you are, the easier you can get along without sleep, but after seventy-two hours of sleep loss most people will have troubles regardless of age. The record for going without sleep is held by a disc jockey who, in a contest, managed to remain sleepless for two hundred sixty-nine hours. However, at the end of that time, he had to be hospitalized for a condition of extreme mental deterioration. To summarize, there are certain limits now established, such as at least four hours sleep per twenty-four hours and no more than seventy-two hours without sleep. But within those broad limits, the particular pattern of sleep that is best for you can only be determined by trial and error. There is no single magic number of hours of sleep that is good for everyone.

▶▶▶ BRAIN MECHANISMS OF SLEEP

We now know some of the mechanisms in the brain that control sleep. In an area about where the neck joins the head is the sleep center of the brain. It is a group of specialized nerve cells. This part of the brain controls sleep. Drugs that cause sleep, and those that cause excitement and wakefulness, act on this part of the brain. Drugs that cause sleep work one of two ways on these nerve cells. First, a drug may directly cause sleep by slowing the actions of the cells in the sleep center. A number of the common sedative drugs act this way. Second, some drugs produce sleep less directly. They block action of nerve fibers that enter into the sleep center from sensory organs such as the eyes and the ears. By blocking these nerve fibers from the sensory nerve paths to the sleep center, the drugs cause the brain to stop being excited by the input from these sense organs. Thus, sleep comes because of a lowered attention to stimuli in the environment.

Hypnotics

The drugs that directly produce sleep have a number of common properties. These drugs are called "hypnotics" and are the ones that you would most likely receive by prescription for insomnia. Alcohol is one hypnotic drug you can get without a prescription. All hypnotic sleeping drugs are very much alike. The actions of all hypnotic drugs are additive if you take more than one at a time. So, if you were to take, for example, a dose of a barbiturate sleeping pill and two ounces of alcohol, you'd get an additive effect of the two. They both directly reduce the activity of the nerves of your sleep center. The combination of two drugs acting on the same part of the brain causes an effect equal to that of taking twice as much of either alone. The same principle applies to any other combination of hypnotic drugs.

Alcohol

Alcohol is the most common hypnotic drug. It is also, by far, the oldest. By 1000 B.C., the Egyptians had already developed wines and beers. Probably, beers were in common use long before this time. Alcohol has been produced in almost every known culture, in every known time in history. I recently found out that even as deprived a group as the primitive Eskimos had managed to find a way to get alcohol. It is said that an Eskimo would find a bear, follow it until it ate grass, then would kill the bear, cut its stomach out and tie both ends. Then he would wait until the enzymes and acids in the bear's stomach fermented the grass. By this process, the Eskimo would obtain an alcohol-containing beverage, which must have tasted terrible. However, man seems willing to do almost anything to get drunk occasionally. It seems that consuming drugs that will intoxicate, cause the condition of confusion and conceit characteristic of intoxication, is one of the features that distinguishes man from animals. Man is the only animal that voluntarily gets drunk without special training.

Alcohol affects the body in a number of ways besides causing intoxication followed by sleep. Its action slows not only the part of the brain that produces sleep, but also the breathing system, producing death if an overdose is taken. However, seldom does respiratory slowing due to alcohol, by itself, cause death. This may be because the drinker usually does something foolish enough to kill himself another way first. Common causes of death for drunks are auto accidents, falls, and freezing.

Concerning the dose-response effects of alcohol, it takes approximately 2 ounces to induce mild intoxication, 6 ounces to induce definite intoxication, over 6 ounces to cause obligatory sleep. The therapeutic safety ratio for alcohol is between 1:5 and 1:10. To produce death from respiratory slowing one would have to take approximately 50 to 100 ounces of pure alcohol. When considering the dose-response curve for alcohol you must take into account that amounts are in terms of pure alcohol. The term "proof" describes the alcohol content of various beverages. Proof number is twice the pure alcohol content. For example, a fifty proof beverage contains 25 percent alcohol, a one-hundred-proof beverage contains 50 percent alcohol, and so on.

After ingestion of a quantity of alcohol, there is the phenomenon known as "the hangover." This is characterized by nausea, headache, general feeling of weakness, and a dark brown taste in the mouth. If one consumes between a pint and a quart of alcohol every day and continues to do so for two months to a year, dependence will develop. This is a physical dependence. Upon abrupt withdrawal of a drug a dramatic physiologic upset will result. With alcohol, this withdrawal has been named delirium tremens (DTs) or rum fits. Withdrawal symptoms are severe. Death results in up to 15 percent of the cases where there is an abrupt withdrawal of the drug and no medical treatment available. Both psychological and physiological dependence on alcohol are very strong. The relapse rate for alcoholism is in the neighborhood of 50 to 75 percent of all people who become dependent, even considering all treatment methods known today. It is almost true to say that there is no such thing as an ex-alcoholic — only an alcoholic who hasn't yet relapsed.

There is some development of tolerance to alcohol. Continued taking of alcoholic beverages causes the liver to form more enzymes that detoxify alcohol more rapidly. However, this enzymatic tolerance is not as potent as the "behavioral" tolerance to alcohol. People who are often drunk learn to compensate for the way they act. They walk more slowly, they speak more slowly, and in other similar ways compensate for the behavioral incapacities caused by alcohol.

At this time in the United States, the consumption of the drug alcohol at too high a dose, too often, and for too long a time, is, without a doubt, the most serious drug problem of our society. Approximately one hundred million Americans drink occasionally. Of that number, one in ten will become a "problem" drinker during his or her life. By problem drinker, I do not necessarily mean a person who is dependent upon alcohol. Rather, I mean that alcohol produces problems in the form of jail, divorce, automobile accidents, and so on. That alcohol is our largest drug problem is evidenced by a recent study in a Minnesota city. On a particular day, all the hospitals of the town were surveyed to see how many of the patients were brought in primarily for drug-related problems. Of all patients, 3 percent were there with primarily drug-related disorders, of these 2.1 percent were for alcohol and only 0.9 percent for other drugs. Also, in a study of the corpses of persons who had been involved in lethal automobile accidents in the state of New York, over half had levels of blood alcohol that would have caused drunkenness. Again, 47 percent of all sex crimes in the United States are associated with the use of alcohol; 86 percent of all crimes involving child molesting are alcohol related. When you consider these statistics, I think it's easy to see that the problems associated with the misuse of the drug alcohol outweigh, in sheer magnitude and severity, anything we can conceive of for other drugs. For those who want further data on the insanity or liver disorders that can result from long-term use of alcohol, or the many other problems associated with its use, I refer you to *Alcohol Problems: A Report to the Nation* by Thomas Plaut, Oxford University Press, 1967.

On the other hand, before we say too many bad things about alcohol, note that man has always occasionally sought a state of intoxication. Indeed, an occasional escape from reality, whether by alcohol, television, a vacation, or other means, may even be beneficial for our mental well-being. Alcohol for 90 percent of those who use it does not cause problems. It gives pleasure to them. Further, alcohol is a useful hypnotic drug, particularly for the elderly. A friend of mine who runs a geriatric hospital has given up the use of sleeping pills to help his elderly patients sleep. Instead, he has taken to pushing a cart around, mixing martinis, manhattans, highballs, or whatever the patients might wish. He is using alcohol as a hypnotic drug for these patients. They seem to enjoy it more than pills and it is just as effective and useful. I have begun using beer for some of the patients in a hospital with which I am associated. I have found this to be preferable to sleeping pills, both as a pleasant, socializing event and as a hypnotic drug for many of the patients.

Chloral Hydrate

Another chemical, quite similar to alcohol, that is used as a hypnotic is chloral hydrate (Noctec, Aquachloral, Felsules, Kessodrate) and its derivatives trichloroethanol, petrichloral (Periclor), chloral betaine (Beta-Chlor), trichloroethylphosphate (Triclofos), and chlorobutanol (Chloretone). Chloral hydrate will slow the nerves in the sleep center in the same way alcohol does. Also, both chloral hydrate and alcohol add their effects, so if these drugs are taken together, you get an effect greater than from each taken alone. Finally, if a person is dependent upon alcohol and alcohol is abruptly withdrawn, chloral hydrate will prevent the withdrawal syndrome. These facts indicate that the mechanisms of action of chloral hydrate and of alcohol are similar.

The dose usually used with chloral hydrate is between 1 and 2 gm to induce sleep. The pattern of intoxication followed by sleep is very similar to that of alcohol. Approximately 10 gm of chloral hydrate are lethal. Again, we have a therapeutic safety ratio of about 1:10, the same as with alcohol.

Barbiturates

The most commonly used hypnotic drugs are the derivatives of barbituric acid called barbiturates. You can generally recognize these because almost all of them have trade names that end in "al," such as Luminal, Seconal, Nembutal. This isn't always true, however. The barbiturates are intoxicant drugs that interact with alcohol, as does chloral hydrate, to produce greater effects than when taken alone. They have very similar effects on breathing. They act directly upon the nerves of the sleep center, slowing their activity. Also, barbiturates can be substituted for alcohol to prevent a withdrawal syndrome. Thus, though barbiturates are drugs that can only be obtained by prescription, they are pharmacologically very similar to the common, nonprescription drug alcohol. This is evidence of the occasional lack of relationship between the pharmacological properties of drugs and the laws that govern their use in our society today.

Barbiturates are generally classified in terms of their time-action curves. There are the ultrashort acting barbiturates that act for about twenty minutes, such as thiopental (Pentothal), the short to medium acting barbiturates that act for three to eight hours, such as amobarbital (Amytal), aprobarbital (Alurate), butabarbital (Butisol), pentobarbital (Nembutal), secobarbital (Seconal), and vinbarbital (Delvinal), and the long-acting barbiturates that work for about twelve hours, phenobarbital (Luminal), mephobarbital (Mebaral), and metharbital (Gemonil). The ultrashort acting barbiturates all have to be given by injection, so they are less commonly available. The most used barbiturates are the short– to medium-acting ones. With these, the usual dose prescribed for "sedation," that is, for relaxation without sleep, is 50 mg to 100 mg. The dose generally prescribed for hypnosis, that is, to induce sleep, is 100 mg to 200 mg. At a dose of 300 mg almost everyone will have a period of intoxication followed by fairly profound sleep. The lethal dose, which causes a paralysis of respiration due to its actions on the breathing control center of the lower brain, is about five to ten times the dose necessary to induce sleep. This would be in the range of 500 mg to 1500 mg of a short-acting barbiturate all taken at one time.

The long-acting barbiturates are not often used to induce sleep but are generally used to produce sedation and muscular relaxation. Phenobarbital is the most common one. They are usually given at a dose not to exceed 50 mg in a day. Phenobarbital has one additional use that is different from other barbiturates. It is an effective anticonvulsant. It is used for people who have convulsions due to epilepsy or other neural disorders. Phenobarbital, in a low dose, is a standard drug used to control these disorders. Although there are many new drugs for control of epilepsy, phenobarbital is often still the drug of choice. More will be said on this topic in a later chapter.

All of the barbiturates cause a period of depressed mental functioning, both during their action and following their use. Their "aftereffect" is sometimes referred to as a barbiturate "hangover." It differs a great deal from the nausea and headache of the alcohol hangover. The person is in a depressed mood, he is slow in muscular performance, and generally feels dragged out. This "hangover" occurs not only during the initial time before a barbiturate induces sleep or during its sedative action, if it is taken at a low dose, but for as long as eighteen hours after the barbiturate has been taken. On the afternoon of the next day, after taking a hypnotic dose of the barbiturate to go to sleep at night, the person will still have some small degree of effect.

Tolerance of the sedating and hypnotic effects of barbiturates develops. You have to take more and more of the drug in order to put yourself to sleep if you take barbiturates for over a week. Unfortunately, tolerance of the drug in the breathing center does not develop as rapidly. Therefore, a person who takes these drugs on a chronic basis must constantly raise the dose to induce sleep while the dose necessary to cause death due to respiratory paralysis remains lower. The therapeutic safety ratio would start as 1:5 or 1:10, but it changes with tolerance to as little as 1:2 or 1:3. This treads a bit close to the edge of danger.

The type of dependence developed with barbiturates is very similar to that formed with alcohol. The symptoms displayed on abrupt withdrawal are almost identical. To achieve a state of physical dependence you must take at least 800 mg to 1,000 mg every day for a few months. As with alcohol, on abrupt cessation of barbiturate use, for one who is physically dependent, the withdrawal can be lethal in about 15 percent of the cases in which withdrawal is attempted without medical supervision.

Barbiturate use has an important effect on society. The barbiturates, either alone or in combination with alcohol, are the drugs that cause the greatest number of accidental deaths due to acute overdose. The standard pattern of this cause of death is as follows: first, the person drinks alcohol to excess, then, in order to get to sleep, takes barbiturate sleeping pills; finally, since both drugs cause intoxication and memory loss, the person forgets he took the sleeping pills and takes more. Death results due to the additive effects of alcohol and barbiturate on the breathing control center. Barbiturates are also a common cause of infant mortality and are second to aspirin as the major cause of accidental death due to drugs in children. Finally, these "downers," the street term for barbiturates, are not without hazard; they are the drugs of choice for suicides in the United States. Another source of potential harm from barbiturates or alcohol is their effect on people who are mentally depressed. These drugs may act to cause some degree of mood depression, both during their initial activity and during the "hangover" period. These possible problems must certainly be taken into consideration if you are using them for their therapeutic effects of muscle relaxation, tranquilization during the day, or sleep at night. You must be aware of the harm that can come when these drugs are misused.

Nonbarbiturate Hypnotics

A new series of hypnotic drugs have entered the market that were believed to be safer than barbiturates. Some people thought that they would have none of the problems associated with the barbiturates. Unfortunately, all of these new hypnotics have the identical problems that the barbiturates have. They can produce physical dependence when taken too often, in too great an amount, for too long. They are additive in their effects with alcohol or barbiturates. They produce mental depression the next day, and their therapeutic safety ratios are about the same as those of the barbiturates. There seems to be little to recommend these newer hypnotic drugs over the older, cheaper barbiturates. These newer drugs are glutethimide (Doriden), which has a usual hypnotic dose of 500 mg; ethinamate (Valmid), usual hypnotic dose 500 mg; methyprylon (Noludar), usual hypnotic dose 200 mg to 400 mg; methaqualone (Quaalude), usual hypnotic dose 150 mg to 300 mg; and the chloral hydrate–like drug, ethchlorvynol (Placidyl), usual hypnotic dose 500 mg.

An exception to these "nonbarbiturate-type" sleeping drugs, which act so much like barbiturates, are two very new drugs that were developed from the benzodiazepine class of tranquilizers (Librium-like). These are nitrazepam (Mogadon) and flurazepam (Dalmane). Far less is known as to why these drugs are able to cause sleep but they do not seem to act the same way as the barbiturates. They do not as directly depress the sleep center and have far less effect upon the respiratory center in the lower brain. For this reason, the therapeutic safety ratio for these drugs is well over 1:100, as opposed to 1:5 or 1:10 for the barbiturates. This means that they will be less likely to be used for suicide, and it will be difficult for a person to accidentally poison himself with one of these drugs. There is some evidence that the following day they do cause a hangover effect. Also, the quality of sleep may be better with these drugs than with barbiturates. We still have much to learn about these benzodiazepine hypnotics. Thus far, there has been no evidence that a physical dependence, of a barbiturate type, can develop with the benzodiazepine hypnotics. They can cause a different, less severe, dependence of their own. However, it takes a very large dose taken over a very long time to produce this dependence. The addition of these new sleeping compounds to our armamentarium of chemicals is very welcome.

Nonprescription Sleeping Pills

Presently there are a number of sleeping pills on the market that can be bought in the supermarket or drugstore without a prescription. They are advertized as being able to "gently induce sleep," and as being "non-habit-forming" and "nonbarbiturate." The sales records of these "sleep aids" is evidence of the great desire of the people in the United States to be awake when they wish to be awake and to be asleep when they wish to be asleep. At one time, man was more or less content to regulate his life by the movement of the earth in relation to the sun. Today everything, from automobiles to television sets, alarm clocks, and factory whistles, requires man to be awake or asleep in response to the tempo of society. Perhaps this is the reason, as well as the general tension that surrounds our lives in a post-industrial society, that causes us to have such a need for sleep-inducing compounds.

The advertising for the nonprescription sleeping pills is true when taken quite literally. They are not habit forming if you mean that physical dependence will not result from their continuous use. However, I think that anything done on a regular basis can be regarded as a habit. So, to say that these drugs are not "habit" forming is really a bit misleading. People do get into the habit of taking these pills night after night. There is no physical withdrawal syndrome when ingestion is discontinued, but many people will get so much in the habit that they cannot sleep without taking these pills. Moreover, when advertisers say they are nonbarbiturate they are also *literally* correct. They are not barbiturates and they do not act to directly slow the sleep center. Rather, they seem to act indirectly either by making the brain itself less receptive to environmental stimuli or by blocking the impulses from the senses to the sleep center.

These sleep aids usually contain a number of drugs. Most of them are combinations of specific sleep-inducing ingredients added to various old folk remedies, even such questionable compounds as extract of passion flower, vitamins, and salicylamide. However, for the most part, there are only two major types of truly active drugs in the sleeping pills that can be obtained without a prescription. These are extracts, or derivatives, of the belladonna plant or synthetic products that resemble them, and antihistamines.

Belladonna Sleeping Pills

The belladonna plant derivative that is most usually found in these sleep aid preparations is scopolamine (hyoscine). It is present sometimes simply in the form of scopolamine, other times in the form of scopolamine aminoxide hydrobromide, or occasionally as a belladonna product called hyoscyamine. It really doesn't matter whether it is in one form or another. Generally, the dose of scopolamine present in sleeping pills will vary between 0.125 mg and 0.6 mg. The precise amount per capsule, of course, will depend upon the number of capsules that you are instructed to take and what other products are present with the scopolamine. Scopolamine at these doses does cause a relaxing effect. The mechanism of this relaxation is not well understood, but it appears to affect the mechanism in your brain that tells you how important environmental stimuli are. In other words, it makes your environment less interesting. This is called a "dissociative" effect. Things just don't turn you on. This allows sleep to occur.

Increasing the dose of this type of drug to a high level does not bring a greater degree of sedative effect. Quite the contrary, you can get an excitation if you increase the dose too high. Further, with very high doses, scopolamine becomes unpleasantly hallucinogenic, that is, it causes nightmarish illusions. The normal side effects of scopolamine at a sedative dose level are dryness in the mouth and nose, occasional dizziness, and sometimes, a ringing in the ears.

Antihistamine Sleeping Pills

The second component found in most nonprescription sleeping pills is one of the antihistamines. Generally this will be methapyrilene, usually at a total dose of 25 mg to 50 mg; pyrilamine maleate, 6 mg to 18 mg; hydroxyzine, 25 mg to 50 mg; or doxylamine at 25 mg to 50 mg. These compounds, also, do not produce a direct slowing of the nerves in the sleep center. The means by which they cause the drowsiness and sleep is not known, but that it is not due to their antihistamine effects is known. A person may get a strong sedating effect from a particular antihistamine and yet get little antihistaminic benefits. Another person might have exactly opposite results from the same antihistamine. Although there is little evidence of tolerance development with scopolamine, this is not true for the antihistamine components of these sleeping pills. For example, methapyrilene loses its ability to induce sleep if it is taken every day for a period of two or three weeks. Taking of a greater quantity of an antihistamine than the recommended dose does not cause any increase in drowsiness. At the recommended dose a ceiling effect is reached. These same antihistamines are added to analgesics and cold remedies.

Both scopolamine and the antihistamines have very high lethal doses, giving a high therapeutic safety ratio, probably in the range of about 1:500 or more. On the other hand, both scopolamine and the antihistamines can produce drug allergies.

Chapter 4

Antiseptics (Disinfectants)

Antiseptics (disinfectants or germicides) are any drugs that you place on your body, gargle, swallow, or use to wash objects in your environment that will kill or stop the growth of germs. They are not supposed to be absorbed into your bloodstream as are antibiotics. By "germs" I mean all the various microorganisms, both large, such as funguses, and small, such as bacteria and viruses.

Germs are not all bad. Some are good. Some are bad. Most are indifferent to your health and well-being. Normally you have an array of various kinds of germs in your mouth, nose, ears, skin, stomach, intestines, and hair. Many of these germs are not bad for you. Many of them are actually good for you. For example, some germs in your intestines aid in the breakdown of fecal material. Without their aid you would be less able to reabsorb water from your gut. This is the reason that when you take some of the antibiotic drugs, you get a runny stool. The antibiotic kills the good germs in your intestine as well as the harmful ones. The result is diarrhea, that is, an inability of your gut to reabsorb water. Another example that shows that not all germs are harmful is the situation of having germs on your skin. You normally have a large complement of various germs on your skin. Most of these germs neither help you nor harm you. They are just there. Thus, you shouldn't get "germophobia." You should be adequately discriminating about the good germs, the bad germs, and those that are of no importance to your health.

▶▶ GENERAL FACTS ABOUT ANTISEPTICS

Different antiseptics can kill many types of germs. However, no particular antiseptic works on all kinds of germs. Some types of germs are highly resistant to antiseptics. Second, antiseptics differ in their ability to get to the site of the infection. Third, to be effective, the antiseptic must be in an adequate concentration to kill or to prevent the growth of the germ colonies at the site of infection. Fourth, they should have as few toxic effects as possible on the cells of the body. Moreover, the goal of having the correct kind of antiseptic activity for the particular type of germ reach the correct area in an adequate concentration and still to be nontoxic is quite difficult to attain. Indeed, most attempts to medicate cuts and wounds by the average person are probably a completely wasted effort. Most people use these antiseptic medications in a ritual manner in solutions, sprays, powders, in their mouths as gargles, in their ears as drops, over their bodies in soaps, in their rectums as suppositories almost without consideration as to what kind of germ they're trying to stop, or even whether it's good to try to get rid of that particular kind of germ. Seldom do these antiseptics penetrate to the level of the germ. Generally, a germ will be deep enough in the skin, under the horny, protein layer that is the surface of the skin, that the antiseptic substance can't get to it. Also, a number of the antiseptics are safe when applied to intact skin, but if they are placed on a wound or a burn, they can be quite toxic since they can enter the bloodstream. So, you see many common uses of antiseptics are useless and some are harmful.

Wound Care

If you have a wound, first cleanse away any debris around it by washing. Then, give the area very thorough rinsing with water. Finally, cover it with a bandage that has perforations to allow air to penetrate. You will now have done about everything you can to eliminate germs. You have achieved just about as much as if you had placed an antiseptic on the area. Beyond this, most infections are only effectively handled by the identification of the specific type of germ and then the use of the correct antibiotic taken internally to get at the germ from the inside.

▶▶ HISTORIC USES OF ANTISEPTICS

The use of antiseptics is ancient. People have been cutting themselves, or each other, since the beginning of recorded history. One of the earliest lessons learned was that if salt water was put on a wound it was a bit less likely to become full of pus, an evidence of infection. However, it was not understood until the time of Lister that a dirty environment was an important factor in infection. Then, with the aid of Koch and Pasteur, the "germ theory" of infection came into existence. We finally realized that we were living with a great many tiny organisms that also inhabited our world.

Our forebears soon recognized that it is far better to prevent an infection, by having a clean environment, than to try to treat the infection once it exists. The ancient Persians required that drinking water be stored in bright copper pots. They didn't know that metallic ions, such as copper, were good antiseptics, but they did find that they lost fewer people from waterborne infections. The ancient use of wine and vinegar to purify water is another example of antiseptic action based on alcohol and acetic acid as germ killers.

We seem to have forgotten the lesson that a clean environment is the best way to avoid infection. Recently there has been an increase of staphylococcal infections in our hospitals. Because of the success of the antibiotic drugs, many hospitals have become very lax in their sanitary procedures. They don't scrub and clean as much as they used to. The result has been an outbreak of a form of staphylococcus that is resistant to the majority of our antibiotics. This has led to the necessity of reconsidering the advantages of scrubbing the rooms with various antiseptic solutions, such as carbolic acid, to keep the population of germs down. Infectious hepatitis is another infection that is easy to prevent but hard to cure. It is a viral infection and is spread by unsanitary living conditions. It can be easily stopped by an efficient use of antiseptics in living areas, by adequate hand-washing, and by sanitary disposal of fecal material. Please note that infectious hepatitis is a completely different disease from serum hepatitis, which I previously discussed. Serum hepatitis usually is transmitted only by an object, such as a needle, that penetrates directly into the bloodstream. On the other hand, infectious hepatitis is passed through foods, kissing, touching, and inadequate sanitation facilities. I hope these examples stress the point that a sanitary environment, produced by washing with soap, water, and antiseptics, is the best approach. Using antiseptics in you or on you is relatively inefficient.

Phenol Antiseptics

One of the oldest and most effective of the antiseptics is phenol (carbolic acid) and its derivatives. Some common derivatives of phenol are cresols, creosote, resorcinol, hexylresorcinol, thymol, parachlorophenol and, perhaps its most famous modern progeny, hexachlorophene. We'll discuss hexachlorophene separately since it has come into a good deal of notoriety recently. Hexachlorophene excepted, the phenols all act in about the same way. Phenols have the ability to kill germs by causing a breakdown of protein. Germs are full of protein. Phenol, at a concentration of as low as 0.2 percent, can stop the growth of germs by its ability to penetrate into the germs and then to cause the breakdown of complex proteins necessary for the life of the germ. At a strength of more than 1 percent, the majority of common germs are killed. At 1.3 percent or above, most funguses will be killed. Phenols have a high degree of efficacy in water, but they are rendered essentially inactive by soap. This points to one rather general problem with the use of antiseptics. After you wash a wound or any object, you'll probably leave some soap residue, no matter how thoroughly you try to rinse. Soap inactivates phenols and a number of the other antiseptics. Thus, you must rinse very thoroughly or use a detergent, not a soap, that doesn't inactivate the antiseptic.

If you examine many of the common commercial antiseptics, you'll find some amount of phenol in them, sometimes at a concentration too low to be effective but, nevertheless, with some phenol. This low concentration of phenol is added because when the drug is applied to the skin in adequate concentration, it causes a breakdown in the protein of the skin as well as in germs, the skin breakdown leaves a white covering, then the area turns red and some skin layers slough off. This leaves the skin surface stained a brown color, but a surface on which the germs are more exposed. Phenol also has the property of being a mild local anesthetic. It will produce a feeling of warmth and tingling. However, generally at a concentration necessary to get the warmth and tingling feeling, or to kill germs, you also kill part of the skin. Thus, when using it to wash objects you should be sure to use rubber gloves. On the other hand, its ability to cause the outside layers of skin to slough off helps it or other antiseptics to get at the germs.

Phenol has a marked action on your central nervous system. It can get into your bloodstream through every possible site of administration, even intact skin. It is easily absorbed. If you have a cut, or it is absorbed through the mucous membrane of your mouth or throat, or even through intact skin, you can get a dose of phenol adequate to cause poisoning. Poisoning by phenol produces a central nervous system stimulation that causes muscle tremor and convulsions. Your blood circulation is depressed so your blood pressure falls. You get very, very cold as it affects the part of your brain controlling temperature regulation. The toxic dose for an oral ingestion of phenol in the adult is between 8 gm and 15 gm. Children and older people are much more sensitive to it. Further, you can build up the phenol level in your blood over a period of time. For these reasons phenol should be used with caution. If you apply it to the skin, get it into a cut, gargle with it, and so on, at a dose that is adequate to produce an antiseptic action to kill germs, you will probably be irritating and killing your tissue, too. If you have it around the house and someone drinks it, or if you place it on too large an area of your body for too long a time, or on an area of your body that is abraded or burned, it can get into your bloodstream. You can then die from phenol poisoning. Thus, there are presently very few legitimate therapeutic uses for phenol. On the other hand, it's a great antiseptic with which to scrub your environment. Just wear rubber gloves and be careful. The derivatives of phenol, cresol, creosote, resorcinol, hexylresorcinol, thymol, and parachlorophenol, are similar in their activities to phenol itself. They differ from it only in their potency, both in toxic effects on your body and toxic effects on germ cells.

Hexachlorophene

Hexachlorophene is a phenol derivative that deserves special mention. It has a number of characteristics that make it more useful than other phenol-type antiseptics. First, it has a less irritating effect on the skin than the other phenols. Also, it has a higher toxicity for certain types of germs and funguses. Finally, it is not inactivated by soap. These characteristics have led to its use for routine washing of infants with hexachlorophene preparations in hospitals to reduce skin infections, and its use in vaginal deodorants for women. Indeed, between three and four hundred different products for almost every use conceivable have been sold until recently when the Food and Drug Administration banned its use except by prescription. Hexachlorophene is now commonly found in the blood of almost every American. Generally, it has been present in blood in the amount of about 0.001 parts per million. However, mouthwash users who gargled once a day with a solution of 0.5 percent hexachlorophene for three weeks built up their blood levels to about 0.06 parts per million. People who used deodorant soaps with hexachlorophene daily built up blood levels to 0.38 parts per million and the twenty-four million American females who used vaginal deodorant sprays or acne sufferers who used soaps or lotions containing hexachlorophene built up to even higher levels. So when you take your next bath, if you still have a deodorant soap with hexachlorophene you must consider the possibility that you are building up high blood levels of this drug. Indeed, you have to build up high levels of hexachlorophene in your blood to get any germ killing effect on your skin. The concentration of hexachlorophene buildup to be effective in killing germs on your skin takes between two to four days of continued use of a deodorant soap. If you take only one shower using a deodorant soap and don't use it again, you have not killed those germs that live on your skin and combine with the organic matter to cause odor. You might as well have used a nonmedicated soap.

If you have a cut or a burn, there will be a greater penetration of hexachlorophene into your body than when used on intact skin. Further, in considering the use in deodorant vaginal sprays, you must realize that the usual types of germs that cause vaginal odors are not killed by hexachlorophene.

To summarize, the good things that can be said about hexachlorophene are that it is not inactivated by soap, and it is effective as an antiseptic in killing many different types of germs. It can effectively reduce body odor if used continuously, and it has proven very effective in the reduction of staphylococcal germ infections in infants in hospitals. On the other hand, hexachlorophene has some large hang-ups. First, it is absorbed into the bloodstream quite easily through the mucous membrane of the mouth or vagina; it is absorbed to some degree by intact skin and will enter the body in large quantities if the skin is broken with a wound or burn. Further, a minute quantity of an impurity which is fairly common as an accidental addition to hexachlorophene preparations is a group of chemicals known as dioxins. Even the most minute amount of these dioxins can cause skin eruptions and acne.

Hexachlorophene is known to have the same sort of effect on the central nervous system as the other phenols. Recent experimentation has shown that a special two-week diet containing added hexachlorophene that would bring a rat to a blood level of 0.9 to 1.5 parts per million caused brain damage. I want to emphasize that the amount of a chemical that will damage a rat is not necessarily the same amount that will damage a man. On the other hand, when I see data like these, it does make me wonder and worry. So, we do know that a quantity of hexachlorophene, in the blood of a rat, that is about three times greater than the amount developed by regular showering with a deodorant soap containing hexachlorophene, is an adequate amount to cause harm to the rat. However, it isn't necessary to throw away all bars of deodorant soap. At this time, no one has shown actual damage to humans due to the use of hexachlorophene soaps, mouthwashes, or sprays on undamaged skin or mucous membrane. There have been reports of difficulties for people who placed hexachlorophene on broken or burned skin. Also, babies are very sensitive to the effects of hexachlorophene. In one study, in which infant monkeys were washed for weeks in a solution like that used for human babies, it was found the monkeys did develop brain damage. For this reason, the amount of washing of babies with hexachlorophene in hospitals has been dramatically reduced. Also, they have been rinsing the babies a great deal more thoroughly. However, to show the other side of the coin, one hospital that completely cut out the use of hexachlorophene began to have outbreaks of skin eruptions due to staphylococcus infection in babies. The hospital went back to the use of hexachlorophene soaps but with a very careful rinsing and with a reduction in the number of washings of the baby.

Alcohol as an Antiseptic

Alcohol has been known for seventy-five years to be an effective antiseptic. It must be placed in a 70 percent solution with water, that is, seven parts of alcohol and three parts of water. Interestingly, at either a higher or lower percentage of alcohol, you have a far less effective antiseptic. Alcohol is also used as a carrier substance in a large number of antiseptic compounds. However, the percentage of alcohol is seldom close to the optimal 70 percent figure. A difficulty with alcohol as an antiseptic is that its activity on germs depends on its ability to cause a breakdown in the outside membrane of a germ cell. When it is applied to sensitive tissues of the human body, that is, mucous membranes, the cells of human tissue also break down in a similar manner. This causes a great deal of irritation. So, when it is placed on an open wound or in your mouth, in an adequate concentration to be antiseptic, alcohol burns your tissue as well as killing the germs.

Boric Acid

Boric acid is a very weak antiseptic. It does not kill cells as much as it stops them from growing in those areas that have been saturated with a boric acid solution. It is nonirritating. This property has made its application to the eye very common, usually as an eye wash or ointment. Also, it is used as an ointment and dusting powder for diaper rash and similar disorders for the same reason.

Why boric acid has achieved its prominent place in medicine is difficult to understand since it is very weak as an antiseptic, and it is not a soothing agent. Many people believe boric acid to be a relatively benign, nontoxic substance. This is not true. Since it is such a common compound in the home, boric acid poisoning cases have become rampant. The lethal dose of boric acid for an adult is about 15 gm to 20 gm; for an infant, 5 gm to 6 gm. If boric acid is used as mouthwash or as an enema, it's quite easily absorbed. It goes through mucous tissue with hardly a pause. You can easily absorb enough to be poisoned by it. Further, boric acid excretion is slow and the body does little to detoxify it. You can accumulate a dangerous amount of it over a period of time. Boric acid can penetrate the skin if you have any eruption, cut, or scraping of your outer layer of skin. Thus, it can penetrate into the bloodstream of an infant if it is used for diaper rash. It enters right through the rash.

The first symptoms of boric acid poisoning are nausea, vomiting, and diarrhea. Then body temperature falls and a rash will break out. Next, headache, restlessness, and weakness occur. Death, if it is going to occur, will happen within about five days.

Iodine

Tincture of iodine, which is iodine dissolved in alcohol, was first used as an antiseptic by a French surgeon in 1839. It was one of the most prevalent methods of treating wounds in the U.S. Civil War. Yet, to this day, we don't know how iodine exerts its antiseptic action.

Iodine in a dilution of 1:200,000 destroys all germs when they are exposed to it for fifteen minutes. It is also effective as a fungicide (i.e., kills funguses), a viracide (i.e., kills viruses), and an amoebacide (i.e., kills simple cell parasites). It is easily dissolved in water as well as in alcohol. The sting caused by an alcohol solution can be eliminated from iodine antiseptics by using a water-soluble form.

Iodine is not nearly as toxic as popular opinion seems to believe. Although there have been some attempted suicides with iodine, very few people ever die from it. Iodine tincture, which contains 2 percent iodine and 2 percent sodium iodide, a salt of iodine, dissolved in alcohol, is the usual form consumed to attempt suicide. Fatalities have occurred when between 30 ml and 250 ml of iodine solution have been ingested. This is really quite a lot. Most of the toxicity of iodine is due to its highly corrosive action on the gastrointestinal system. Thus, the first symptoms of iodine poisoning are vomiting and diarrhea with blood showing in the stool. If there has been a severe enough irritation, with massive damage of the stomach and the intestines, the fluid loss from vomiting and diarrhea can cause shock and death within forty-eight hours. Also, in rare cases, there have been people who have gotten an allergic response to iodine. This allergy shows itself in the usual way as described in Chapter 2. However, of the various antiseptic substances it seems that iodine really is one of the best. It can poison but seldom does. Its only major hang-up is that it turns your skin brown. People seem to object to this.

Hydrogen Peroxide

Hydrogen peroxide is an old, commonly used antiseptic of very feeble activity. Hydrogen Peroxide Solution, USP, contains 3 percent hydrogen peroxide in water. When this solution is applied to your tissue it immediately releases oxygen. Very few germs can live in an environment of high concentrations of oxygen. However, the solution usually does not penetrate below the crusty layer of the skin, so it doesn't reach the really critical area of infection. Also, the oxygen is released all at once from the solution, giving this compound a very temporary activity. Hydrogen peroxide does have the advantage of bubbling when it releases the oxygen. This helps to mechanically clean the wound and that is really about the best thing that can be said for it. Hydrogen peroxide is sometimes used as a mouthwash, but the continued use of this drug causes the development of the small, hairlike growths on your tongue. This "hairy tongue" is somewhat disconcerting, but it will go away as soon as you stop using hydrogen peroxide.

Metal Salt Antiseptics

Numerous salts of metals are used as antiseptics. Of these, the salts of mercury and silver are the most common. Mercury is found as mercuric chloride, yellow mercuric oxide, yellow mercuric oxide ointment, mercury ointment, ammoniated mercury, nitromersol (Metaphen), phenylmercuric acetate (Lorophyn), thimerosal (Merthiolate), and merbromin (Mercurochrome). The actions of mercury compounds seem to be that the mercury ion blocks one of the enzymes that is necessary for the growth of germs. It does not kill the germs but stops their growth. All of these compounds must be regarded as relatively feeble germicides. They don't kill, they just slow growth. Also, they do not seem to be effective at killing funguses, but certain viruses may have their growth stopped by the mercury compounds. At concentrations varying between 1:100,000 and 1:1,000, they can stop the growth of most types of germs.

Mercury poisoning, as most of us are now aware because of worry about mercury in swordfish, is a relatively common event in the United States. Since mercury bichloride is used in diaper rinses and calamine, a mercuric compound is contained in dusting powders, in addition to the antiseptic forms of mercury, there is a lot of mercury in our environment. In the recent past, there was even a greater danger. Mercury can also be ingested in the form of calomel, which was once used as a laxative. Mercury is present in our food, in our air, and in our water. It is a product of industrial civilization. Estimates have been made that one in five hundred children have been exposed to mercury in an amount sufficient to cause some degree of poisoning. Lewis Carroll, who wrote *Alice in Wonderland*, knew that hatters, who used mercury for the production of felt hats, could become "mad as a hatter" due to mercury poisoning.

The signs and symptoms of mercury poisoning depend upon how

much you have received, whether it is a cumulative effect over time, and at what age you receive the drug. In chronic poisoning, the major organs affected are the brain, kidneys, and skin. The symptoms are listlessness, disorganization of thought, redness and swelling in the hands and feet, and a destruction of those cells in the kidney that are responsible for the filtration of urine. Further, it can cause skin eruptions, usually on the hands and feet. In acute mercury poisoning there are vomiting, diarrhea, fever, convulsions and death. It's hard to understand why these toxic mercuric substances are still being used when there are safer and more effective agents.

Various types of silver salts can be used as antiseptics. Silver acts by causing the protein in a germ cell to clump together and settle out, that is, to precipitate. It acts on human body tissue in the same way. Therefore, it is not only an antiseptic but also a caustic. This means it kills superficial skin tissue to form a scab. Silver is highly germicidal. In solution it destroys almost all germs at a concentration of 1:1,000.

Silver Nitrate, USP, is the silver antiseptic you're most likely to encounter. It is occasionally used since it is very effective as an antiseptic. Also, its action can be immediately stopped by washing the area with salt solution. This helps control its action. However, since silver salts stain the skin black, people tend not to like this particular treatment. These salts lay down silver on the skin just as they do on a photographic negative. The stain will slowly disappear spontaneously, but it takes quite a while.

Routinely, silver salts are used in the eyes of newborn infants as a preventive of eye diseases. Many states require a 1 percent silver nitrate solution for newborn babies' eyes. It is very effective in clearing infants' eyes of any germs. It is also used to close wounds, since it will form a clot, and for the removal of warts.

Surface-Acting Antiseptics

A new group of antiseptics are the surface-acting agents. These are benzalkonium chloride, benzethonium chloride, methylbenzethonium chloride, tyrothricin, and cetylpyridinium chloride. These drugs are found in everything from cough drops and mouthwashes to antiseptic creams to contraceptive foams. They have the ability to precipitate and to break up the protein in a germ cell. By this mechanism they destroy it. They have a very low toxicity in humans and are relatively nonirritating to tissue. They kill a large number of different kinds of germs. They have many very useful properties. Unfortunately, as is always true, nothing is ever quite as good as it ought to be. First, these agents are inactivated by soap. Second, they are easily absorbed by cotton, rubber, and almost any other porous material. This means that a bandage can pull the material away from the skin. Third, sometimes they form a layer over the skin, their active properties being directed toward the outside. The germs can multiply under this layer, and the layer can prevent other antiseptics from getting through to the germs. Fourth, their antiseptic properties are adversely affected by calcium, magnesium, iron, and aluminum. Thus, many types of dusting powders inactivate them. Finally, the exact degree of acidity of the skin area has a large influence on their efficiency as antiseptics.

The most common use of surface-acting substances that you will probably run into is in mouthwashes or throat lozenges. So, we must consider what causes bad breath. Bad breath generally has its origin from three sources: an upset stomach, the presence of decaying food particles caught in teeth, and disease of gums or teeth. Obviously an antiseptic will do little good for the odors from an upset stomach, and any compound that is gargled and then spit out will have little long-term effect on a disease of the gums or teeth. This leaves us with food particles stuck in the mouth. If you adequately brush your teeth and use dental floss, there should be little food material left in your mouth. Whatever food is left can be rinsed away and spat out with plain water. Finally, if there are any food particles left for germs to work on, the question is whether the surface-acting drugs can get to them in an adequate concentration. These compounds work by precipitating protein. The cells in your mouth contain protein. So these compounds are partly absorbed and deactivated by the mucous tissue of your mouth. Also, saliva reduces the effectiveness of these drugs. Finally, if you have diluted a mouthwash, you may have destroyed any antiseptic efficacy that it had. Studies have shown that if a surface-acting-type mouthwash is taken straight or at a 75 percent concentration, it may have some antigerm activity. But if you have diluted it with water below this concentration, there is a very rapid loss of antiseptic action. On the other hand, mouthwashes containing surface-acting compounds seem to be reasonably safe since they have such a low toxicity and do not irritate the skin. I suppose I think that you should pick out a mouthwash like a perfume. Get one that you like if it gives you confidence. But don't expect it to take the place of proper oral hygiene in the form of tooth-brushing and the use of dental floss followed by the careful rinsing of the mouth with water. Also, there is no evidence that any mouthwash can reduce the number of upper respiratory infections, that is, "colds," or reduce their severity.

Miscellaneous Antiseptics

There is a large group of antiseptic agents not often seen; I will list the names so that you can look them up if you ever need to. They are nitrofurantoin (Furadantin, Macrodantin), nitrofurazone (Furacin), furazolidone (Furoxone), Evans blue dye, phenazopyridine (Pyridium), acriflavine, fluorescein, phenolphthalein, gentian violet, sulfur, anthralin, and balsam. Each of these compounds has its own particular properties but is not in common enough usage these days to discuss in detail.

Two other antiseptics should be mentioned because their principal use is not to kill germs but to stop fungus infections such as athlete's foot. These are undecylenic acid and tolnaftate, which will be discussed in more detail later. These two drugs, plus a variety of other, less active compounds such as propionic acid, sodium propionate, sodium caprylate, benzoic acid, boric acid, salicylic acid, propylparaben, aluminum acetate, aluminum potassium sulfate acetone, bismuth crystal violet, dimethyzole dihydrochloride, diathenaminyl, phenol, fuscian, sodium thiosulfate, potassium permanganate, resorcinol, and thymol, are found in most of the common athlete's foot remedies. Many of these compounds, such as the phenol, thymol, benzoic acid, salicylic acid, potassium permanganate, fuscian, are not very useful as antiseptics but are present because they have the ability to keratolize the skin. Keratolizing the skin means that the protein layer of the outer, crusty portion of the skin is sloughed off. This sloughing of the exterior skin layer makes the site of the infection more accessible to other, potent antiseptics. The best general advice in terms of athlete's foot is to prevent it. An ounce of prevention is worth a ton of cure in this kind of situation. Keep clean, use drying powder in your socks and shoes, don't spread the infection by picking at the lesions between toes, and, if possible, avoid those areas, such as showers and dressing rooms, where funguses are likely to be.

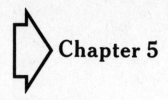

Chapter 5

Stimulants

Stimulant drugs are perhaps consumed more often, without realizing that they are drugs, than any other chemicals. In the United States, a billion kilograms of coffee are consumed each year. Few people realize that the cup of coffee they drink in the morning, or for some, the coffee they drink all day long, is not drunk for its nutritional benefit but because it contains the mood-altering, stimulant-drug caffeine. Also, people who don't drink coffee, but do drink tea, don't realize that tea contains two stimulants, caffeine and theophylline. Perhaps drinkers of cocoa don't know that this drink, which comes from the seeds of theobroma cacao, contains caffeine and theobromine, both of which are stimulant drugs. Again, the cola nuts, which are used to make cola-flavored drinks, also contain caffeine. When you do face these facts, it becomes apparent that the consumption of stimulant, mood-altering drugs is a very common and accepted practice in the United States.

Where the first use of these stimulant drugs, caffeine, theophylline, and theobromine, occurred is lost in the myths of history. However, there is a story that a prior at an Arabian monastery was told by shepherds that goats that ate the berries of the coffee plant gamboled and frisked all night instead of sleeping. The prior, mindful of the long vigils and prayers he had to endure, instructed the shepherds to pick some berries. From these he made a beverage. After drinking the beverage he was not only able to stay awake but even began to enjoy the long night vigils.

▶▶▶ XANTHINE STIMULANTS

Caffeine, theophylline, and theobromine share a number of common therapeutic properties. They all act on the central nervous system to produce stimulation and on the kidneys to produce a copious flow of urine, they stimulate heart muscles and relax smooth muscles, particularly those of the wind pipe. Of the three, caffeine is the most powerful central nervous system stimulant. Theophylline is somewhat less potent but still has marked activities as a stimulant. Theobromine, found in cocoa along with caffeine, has relatively little nervous system stimulating effect. Since these three chemicals are very similar, other than the potency of their effect on the central nervous system, I will refer to them jointly as xanthine stimulants.

The usual oral therapeutic dose of a xanthine for stimulation of the nervous system to cause a mild excitation throughout the brain is between 150 mg and 300 mg. This is the amount found in one or two cups of the average coffee or in about one bottle of a cola drink. When you drink a cup or two of coffee in the morning or have a cola drink, you are drinking the usual therapeutic dose of a xanthine.

A toxic dose of caffeine is about 10 gm. This would be the amount found in between seventy to one hundred cups of coffee. The lethal doses of theophylline and theobromine in man are not known. Some people who drink a great deal of coffee have a mild set of unpleasant reactions characterized by jitteriness, inability to sleep, occasional extra heartbeats, and feelings of tension and unpleasantness.

Recent studies have suggested that coffee drinkers are born, not made. The evidence indicates that some people use large amounts of xanthines but do not have any unpleasant effects. Other people, with even low doses, get unpleasant side effects. These people never seem to be able to enjoy xanthine beverages. They can't even learn to. It may be that they are genetically different from people who can enjoy coffee and other xanthine drinks. This shows that it is necessary always to consider individual differences in reaction to drugs. We are chemically individualistic. Different people can get different effects from the same dose of the same drug.

Caffeine and theophylline reduce the size of the arteries in your brain. It's been shown that there is a decrease in the uptake of oxygen in your brain with a marked reduction of brain blood flow following their ingestion. This may be why xanthines can provide striking relief from a headache caused by high blood pressure. This relief only occurs if the headache is caused by high blood pressure in the brain. The xanthines do not have any analgesic effectiveness for any type of pain other than a high blood pressure headache. They are even antagonistic to the analgesic actions of some of the other drugs. Their use in combination with aspirin and phenacetin, as in APC capsules or other pain medications, is highly questionable.

Although the xanthines constrict the blood vessels in the brain, they dilate the blood vessels of the heart and the skeletal muscles. For this reason they augment heart function. This can be lifesaving in some types of heart failure. Theophylline has become the drug of choice for some patients whose heart blood vessels have become blocked or whose heart action is weak. The increase in blood flow to muscles, due to a dilation of the blood vessels, can increase your capacity for muscular work. They provide a reduction in feelings of fatigue by stimulating your brain and, at the same time, cause an increase of blood flow to your muscles that can help you actually accomplish more work.

The xanthines also act on the stomach by an indirect mechanism. Xanthines cause an increased flow of hydrochloric acid and the enzyme pepsin, which jointly are responsible for the digestion of food in the stomach. Because of this action, xanthines can be a problem if you are predisposed to hyperacidity or if you have an ulcer. Most persons who have ulcers or tendencies toward stomach hyperacidity should be discouraged from an excessive use of any products containing xanthines.

Tolerance can develop to a considerable degree for many of the effects of xanthines. This holds particularly for the increased urine output. There is also some degree of tolerance established for the nervous-system-stimulating properties, but this is not nearly as marked as the tolerance that is developed to the effects on the kidneys.

Dependence on xanthines can develop. This is characterized by a caffeine-withdrawal headache and nervousness in people who have consumed large quantities of xanthines for a considerable period of time who then abruptly stop such drug use. These symptoms of physiological upset caused by the cessation of drug taking reflect physical dependence similar to that on alcohol, barbiturates, or opiates. However, in the case of xanthines, the headache is not so severe nor the craving for the drug so marked as to merit the degree of concern caused by physical dependences produced by other drugs. A psychological dependence on xanthines is certainly developed, but since there is no general social disapproval of the stimulation produced by coffee, tea, or cola drinks, people are not punished for seeking the excitement and mood improvement provided by these drugs.

The mechanism by which xanthines work was discovered recently by Nobel Prize winner E. W. Sutherland. He found that the xanthines affect one of the most fundamental energy-producing mechanisms of the body. The body burns fuels to build a special high-energy chemical to get energy. The xanthines protect these high-energy chemicals from breakdown into other chemicals that would not yield as high an energy level to the body. It is interesting to note that xanthine beverages that have been used for thousands of years have become understood only in the last few years.

Theophylline, or its derivative aminophylline, causes a relaxation in the smooth muscles that surround the air passages in the throat and lungs. This helps to open the airways to allow a freer passage of air. This property has made it useful for disorders such as asthma, chronic bronchitis, and to a limited extent, emphysema. It also increases blood flow to the heart and lungs as well as increasing the rate and force of heart action. It is usually administered at a dose of about 100 mg to 500 mg every four hours. Its most common side effect is gastrointestinal upset. This occurs in 5 percent to 15 percent of patients who take it. The drug can be administered as a pill, as an elixir, as a suppository, or in an aerosol as an inhalant. Each of these forms of administration has some problems. Users should consult their pharmacist about the alternate routes of administration.

▶▶▶ COCAINE-TYPE STIMULANTS

A second type of stimulant drug comes from various derivatives of cocaine (coke, snow) and cocaine-like chemicals. The oldest of these compounds is cocaine itself. Cocaine comes from the leaf of the South American coca plant. For centuries the natives knew that if you combine coca leaf with lime and then chew it, it will allay hunger pangs, make you feel better, and give you a greater capacity for work. This is still a common practice among the natives throughout South America. When a man is drafted into the Peruvian Army, he is told he must cease coca leaf chewing. He does so promptly, since the punishments for continuing are exceedingly severe. Since there is no physical dependence on this drug, he shows no withdrawal signs. He does not chew coca leaves throughout his period in the army. For one reason, he is fed better than he had been as a civilian. Thus, he does not need to allay hunger pangs. When he is discharged from the army, he will again be ill-fed, have to work hard, have little to relieve the boredom and misery of his life, so he will resume chewing coca leaf. From this description you can understand some of the properties of the cocaine that the South American native extracts, in his primitive way, from coca leaf. Cocaine is used to overcome fatigue and to stimulate physical and mental processes. It causes a sense of well-being, a high degree of activity, and a sense of extra energy. Cocaine diminishes hunger pangs.

Cocaine is effective at doses as low as 5 mg to 10 mg. The lethal dose is difficult to establish because people vary tremendously in their individual sensitivity to the drug and also because tolerance develops, not only of the stimulating qualities of cocaine but also of its lethal effects. The approximate lethal dose is 1.2 gm to 1.5 gm. Unpleasant effects can occur at doses as low as 20 mg in some people. The symptoms of cocaine poisoning are restlessness, excitation, and anxiety. Headache is common and a chill may herald the onset of a sudden rise in temperature. Death occurs with an excessively high temperature, accompanied by dilated pupils, nausea, vomiting, finally convulsions and cessation of breathing. It's a rapidly acting drug. After taking a very high dose, death can occur in thirty or forty minutes.

As well as being a stimulant, cocaine has the ability to act as a surface anesthetic. It is a powerful anesthetic agent when placed in the eye and on or under the skin. This property will be discussed further in the chapter on analgesics. Cocaine produces an extreme constriction of the blood vessels of mucous membranes. For this reason, people who have sniffed cocaine sometimes have such a severe constriction of the blood vessels in their nose that the tissue in the nose dies. Repeated use can produce a hole through the central septum of the nose. Years ago, a hole through the septum of regular cocaine users, from one nostril to the other, was quite a common finding.

Stimulant drugs that are very similar in action to cocaine are the amphetamines such as methylamphetamine (Syndrox, Norodin, Desoxyn, Fetamin), dextroamphetamine (Dexedrine), *dl*-amphetamine (Benzedrine), phenmetrazine (Preludin), benzphetamine (Didrex), phentermine (Ionamin, Fastin), diethylpropion (Tenuate, Tepanil), phendimetrazine (Plegine), and methylphenidate (Ritalin). These drugs have many properties in common with cocaine. They all cause feelings of well-being and central stimulation. They reduce hunger pangs. They increase the ability to perform muscular work by masking fatigue. They cause a rise in body temperature. They are rapidly tolerated. Within as little as three to six days of constant use there is a necessity for a very high dose to obtain the desired effects. They do not form a physical dependence. There are no physical withdrawal symptoms on termination of drug taking. They all produce psychic dependence since some people enjoy the feelings of well-being and mental excitation that they cause.

Cocaine and all of these cocaine-like drugs act by causing a release of a hormone called norepinephrine from sites in your brain where it is stored. They also block the re-uptake of norepinephrine into storage sites after it has been released. This release of norepinephrine and the inhibition of its re-uptake causes a greater quantity of free norepinephrine to be present in the brain. It is then available to act upon those parts of the brain that are stimulated by it. The brain centers that are sensitive to norepinephrine stimulate your nervous system to cause a release of other hormones in your body and to produce a general feeling of stimulation and well-being. These drugs work through a very natural mechanism. If you are excited by life events, you naturally cause the release of the chemical norepinephrine from your brain cells. This, in turn, will result in your feeling stimulated. These drugs work through this natural brain mechanism to enhance the amount of the norepinephrine available in your brain. In a sense, the "high" you can get from an exciting skiing trip is a physiological reaction similar to the "high" you could get from cocaine, or drugs similar to cocaine. However, the drug-induced reaction can be a much more intense experience than that caused by skiing if you take a high enough dose. At a moderate dose, the experiences could be equally intense.

Use of Cocaine-like Drugs

Much has been said about the potential benefits and dangers of drugs of this class. People take amphetamines for reduction of appetite to achieve a weight loss. If weight is lost and stays reduced this can be beneficial to health. Overweight is one of the major causes of high blood pressure. On the other hand, these drugs are quickly tolerated so their effectiveness in weight reduction will be of limited value unless their use is coupled with a good deal of will power. Most people who have tried these drugs in weight reducing programs find that as soon as they quit taking the drugs, they put the weight back on. On the other hand, the drug could be useful as an adjunct in the initial phase of a carefully planned diet program.

The amphetamines have been used for problems of excessive fatigue and boredom. On the other hand, again, because of tolerance buildup, there usually has to be an ever-increasing dose of the drug to yield the desired effect. This dose problem can be controlled, however, by strict adherence to a dosage regime of no more than about 15 mg per day. This type of dose control can minimize the degree of tolerance developed.

A new use of the amphetamines, for children who suffer from hyperkinesis, has caused much controversy. Hyperkinetic children cannot focus their attention on any one thing. They must be constantly moving around, darting here and there, looking in different places. A certain percentage of these children will benefit from treatment with a low dose of amphetamine or of methylphenidate. Not all, but some. Within two weeks of drug administration at an adequate dose (perhaps up to 40 mg per day of amphetamine), it will be clear whether a particular child will or will not be benefited. Children who do obtain benefit, show so marked an improvement in concentration span, patience, and general social adjustment that it is almost miraculous. When children respond by overstimulation, administration of amphetamines can be stopped immediately.

Amphetamines are sometimes used in combination with sedatives or sedating antihistamines to reduce the sedative effects. This type of mixture of a stimulant with a sedative produces a mild feeling of well-being, and it seems to be useful for some people who have unhappy and dull lives. This is the basis of such drug combinations as methylamphetamine plus phenobarbital (Ambar), dextroamphetamine plus amobarbital (Amodex, Anorexin, Appenil, Bludex, Dexamyl, Dexaspan, Meditrol), and many others. Finally, amphetamines have been shown to be able to raise the potency of narcotic analgesics, for example, morphine, codeine, or anileridine, while, simultaneously, eliminating many of their undesired effects, such as sedation, lowered blood pressure, and slow breathing.

Misuse of Cocaine-like Drugs

These stimulants used in moderation can provide help for people, whereas when used in excess, without carefully watching the dosage regimen, they can cause serious problems. The major problem with all the cocaine-like drugs is excessive use or overdose. As an example, let us consider methylamphetamine misuse. Methylamphetamine is known by the "street name" of "speed" or "Meth." The slogan "speed kills" has become known all over our society. Yet, there is little documented evidence that many people have died from overdoses of methylamphetamine, with the possible exception of a few who have indulged in highly competitive athletic endeavors while taking methylamphetamine and then died of either heat prostration or high blood pressure. The phrase "speed kills," used mostly by LSD users, or "acid heads," does not necessarily apply literally. There is evidence that by continually overdosing with methylamphetamine, a so-called "speed freak" can take a gram of the material in pure crystalline form intravenously without dying. Tolerance for these drugs is immense. However, the prolonged sleep loss, combined with the high drug doses, can produce a form of mental disturbance, closely resembling paranoid schizophrenia, in which the person has delusions of grandeur and of persecution and is very forgetful. Rarely, he can become aggressively violent. Then, upon cessation of taking the drug, he will have a period of profound depression. This is the "crash." However, these are troubles that occur only after very large doses of drug, for example, exceeding 80 mg per day of methylamphetamine for a period of at least three days. It is difficult to understand the origin of the widespread reputation of these drugs as causes of antisocial behavior or death. There seems to be little evidence that this occurs except under unusual circumstances. On the contrary, users of "speed," at least during the first two days of their binges, are animated, in a good mood, interested, sometimes too focused on one thing, but do not seem to be dangerous or antisocial. During the last day of a binge when the paranoia is developing, there may be some manifestations of antisocial behavior, but it tends to be a nondestructive sort. Suicides may take place during the depression following an amphetamine trip, but you must take into account the usual user is young and that adolescents are the second most prone group to suicide in the United States — the elderly being the most suicide prone. In the last ten years, we have had a 200 percent increase in adolescent suicides among non-drug-using adolescents. Therefore, whether a suicide is caused by the use of a drug or is caused by society or the acts of friends or parents of a young person is difficult to determine in any specific case.

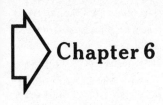

Chapter 6

Stomach Drugs

Most people, at one time or another, will take drugs to relieve indigestion, reduce pain from a peptic ulcer, induce a bowel movement, stop diarrhea, or reduce nausea. Episodic use of antacids, antinauseant compounds, laxatives, or antidiarrhea drugs can help a lot. However, recently, perhaps mostly due to advertising on television and in other mass media, there has been tremendous overemphasis on the necessity for regularity of bowel movements and for the relief of upset due to heartburn. The recent creation of the so-called "blahs" is an example of the mass media producing disorders rather than instructing people in how to cure them. Stomach drugs have become the most often misused and overused drugs we have in our medicine cabinets. In 1968, the sale of antacid compounds alone amounted to 99.3 million dollars. In 1969, the public spent 192 million dollars for laxatives purchased without a prescription. Yet, only 0.6 percent of all prescriptions written by doctors were for laxatives. This indicates that the public is taking laxatives, antacids, and other stomach drugs at a fantastic rate, whereas physicians regard them as drugs that rarely should be taken.

The public seems to regard antacids, laxatives, and similar types of substances for the intestines and stomach as harmless chemicals that can be taken with impunity. This is no more true for stomach drugs than it is for any other drug. There is no such thing as a totally safe drug. Any drug can be misused or overused to an extent that it can be harmful to the person who is using it. On the other hand, I occasionally take antacids when I have an upset stomach or excessive gas. I don't feel that I've been hurt too badly by using antacids in this way, so far. When I'm traveling, I occasionally take laxatives. However, I know that in using drugs in both of these cases I'm probably wasting my money. I probably could have gotten along just as well without the drugs. I, too, have been propagandized by all the mass media ads. Perhaps this is an example that knowledge about drugs does not always guarantee you will use them with wisdom on yourself.

In considering these drugs, it is important for you to realize that many of the things that take place in your intestines and stomach are due to the attitudes that you hold in your head. Your guts are directly sensitive to changes in your emotional state or mood. For that matter, at the dosages commonly used, many of the usual stomach drugs probably have most of their effect on your mind and not your stomach. They cause a "placebo" reaction. A placebo reaction is an effect gained when you believe you are taking an effective drug, but actually the dose is too low or the drug itself is ineffective. You get the effect because you expect it, not because of any chemical action of the drug. It is a very common finding in pharmacology that the expectation of the person taking the drug has a large effect on the outcome of drug action. If you think something is going to make you feel better, the odds are pretty good that it will, particularly if your disorder is affected by your mood.

▶▶▶ REGULARITY OF BOWEL MOVEMENTS

The intensity of advertising has caused an amazing amount of drug use by people to try to ensure "regularity" of bowel movements. Somehow, in our minds, being "regular," whatever that may mean, has become equated with virtue. The fact is that "regularity" is an ill-defined concept. Different people have different patterns of bowel movements. One person might have two bowel movements a day; someone else might have a bowel movement only every three or four days. You might even switch from time to time, sometimes having two or three bowel movements a day or sometimes waiting three or four days to have one. It really doesn't matter. As far as your body is concerned, it doesn't make any difference how often you do it, or whether you switch back and forth. Your bowel is perfectly capable of handling the amount of fecal material that can accumulate in three or four days. Indeed, it is capable of handling a great deal more. In the Arctic, if you're camping under conditions of forty degrees below zero, it is common to undergo voluntary constipation for periods up to three weeks. The option of going out and getting frostbitten buttocks is less pleasant than going without a bowel movement. In this situation, people go without bowel movements for prolonged periods with no ill effects. From this, I think you can see that you shouldn't worry too much about your bowel movements. Let your body take care of itself. If you're taking a laxative more often than once a week, you are probably wasting your money. You may even be hurting yourself by covering up a serious medical disorder for which you should be receiving treatment.

The same reasoning applies to people who are particularly concerned about the texture, color, and consistency of their fecal material. It mostly depends upon your diet. Therefore, as you eat different kinds of foods, there will naturally be a different color, consistency, or texture to your fecal material. It is perfectly all right for it to change. It makes sense that it should change, considering it is the residues from different foods. I'm sure all of us have had the experience of eating beets and having a red tint to our fecal material. Perhaps the best way to avoid becoming concerned about the color, texture, and consistency of your fecal material is not to look at it. The only reason to look at your fecal material is to see if there is any blood in it. If your stool has become black and tarry from bleeding, it can be an important danger sign. If this happens, see your physician at once.

I suppose the moral to this whole story is that, in my opinion, most people are too concerned about their stomachs and intestines. If they would ignore their stomachs and intestines, I think their bodies would generally take care of themselves. If you do, however, encounter problems with an inability to defecate or have a constant soreness or pressure in your stomach, you certainly should see a physician. It is possible that it could be due to heart trouble, gallstones, hernia of the tube connecting your throat to your stomach, troubles in your pancreas, or even, possibly, cancer.

▶▶▶ ANTACIDS

The only medical condition for which antacids are prescribed is the treatment of peptic ulcers. However, most of us occasionally use antacids for various types of stomach distress, with causes ranging from improper eating to excessive alcohol intake. Antacids can be classified into two types: absorbable antacids and those that cannot be absorbed into the blood system.

Absorbable Antacids

The most common absorbable antacid is sodium bicarbonate. Its usual therapeutic dose is about 4 gm. It rapidly and effectively lowers the acidity of the stomach. It also produces carbon dioxide, which aids in the reduction of stomach distress by causing you to belch. Sodium bicarbonate is a cheap, rapid, and effective means of lowering the acidity of the stomach. However, along with all other absorbable antacids, it can cause problems. At its usual therapeutic dose of 4 gm, if you take sodium bicarbonate on a daily basis or more often for a period of time, its absorption into your blood can cause a lowering of the acidity of your blood as well as of your stomach. This lowered acidity of the blood can produce symptoms of hyperirritability, kidney stone, and, if it is very severe, can cause death. A second problem is the buildup of excessive amounts of sodium in the blood. Not only does the bicarbonate get into the blood, but so also does the sodium of sodium bicarbonate. This is a particularly dangerous condition for the elderly or for people on a restricted salt diet. Also, the continued use of an antacid of the sodium bicarbonate type can cause the stomach to secrete more acid. This is the so-called "acid rebound" effect. Finally, although it acts very rapidly, that is, in five to fifteen minutes, its effects go away rapidly also. Its effects seldom last longer than forty-five minutes. The dangers of sodium bicarbonate use seem to outweigh its advantage as a cheap drug.

Nonabsorbable Antacids

Some of the nonabsorbable antacids are calcium carbonate, aluminum hydroxide, magnesium trisilicate, dihydroxy aluminum aminoacetate, magnesium carbonate, and magnesium hydroxide. Of these, calcium carbonate seems to have the greatest effectiveness in rapidly reducing excessive acidity in the stomach. Its usual dose range is between 4 gm and 8 gm. One of its greatest advantages over other nonabsorbable antacids is that it produces neither constipation nor diarrhea.

Magnesium hydroxide (milk of magnesia) is a very popular antacid. Its predominant advantage over others is that it is practically insoluble in water but reacts with the hydrochloric acid in the stomach to form magnesium chloride. The unused magnesium hydroxide remains in the stomach to react with more of the acid as it is formed. It has the longest action of the various antacids. The disadvantages of magnesium hydroxide, or any compound containing magnesium, is that magnesium causes diarrhea. A similar compound is magnesium trisilicate. This is a fairly common ingredient in many commercial antacids. It has the slowest onset, generally taking at least fifteen minutes to start its action. Only 60 percent of its effect is attained in the first hour. However, it has the advantage of not sensitizing the stomach to produce an acid rebound. It, as with other magnesium compounds, produces diarrhea.

Aluminum hydroxide and various other aluminum compounds are also used to lower stomach acidity. Each of these is relatively effective and is not absorbed into the blood. All of the aluminum compounds tend to produce constipation rather than the diarrhea of magnesium compounds.

Most of the tablets available for reduction of stomach acids are mixtures of various antacid drugs. The attempt is usually made to mix an aluminum type antacid with a magnesium one with the hope that the constipation caused by the aluminum compounds will balance the diarrhea caused by the magnesium ones. However, each individual has a different sensitivity to magnesium and aluminum compounds. Therefore, the chance is small that a manufacturer, using a fixed dose of each type of antacid, can hit your particular sensitivities to exactly balance these two effects. You may have to try to find the particular mixture that has just the right percentage of an aluminum and of a magnesium antacid so that you can balance the constipating or diarrhea inducing actions.

In most of the commercially obtainable antacids there will also be a number of other substances present. For example, simethicone is often added to aid in breaking up gas bubbles in the stomach. This facilitates belching for the relief of gas pressure. Other drugs often added are citric acid, glycerin, mint, oil of wintergreen, oil of peppermint, skimmed milk, aluminum phosphate. These do not markedly aid the antacid action but do tend to make the compound more palatable or give it an additional effect of aiding in reducing gas pressure.

The chronic use of antacids of the nonabsorbable type has been associated with very few severe physical problems. This is quite fortunate considering the amounts of these drugs that are taken each year. For the most part, the greatest harm that these compounds do is to your pocketbook, not to your body. However, there have been reports of patients who have had considerable troubles. For example, one person consumed one roll of a popular calcium carbonate antacid per day for over four years. The patient developed calcium deposits in his eyes and in other tissues. He had excessively lowered acidity of his blood, and some degree of misfunctioning in the kidneys. Withdrawal of the drug and a high fluid intake reversed the condition quickly. In another case, with an antacid containing silicone, a person who had been taking thirty to thirty-five tablets a day for two or three years, had kidney stones in which silicone was present. This would indicate that the silicone may have contributed to the formation of the kidney stones. Still, with only these few cases reported, we may conclude that the greatest single problem associated with taking antacids is the absorption of sodium from the absorbable antacids. This is certainly a danger for people who have high blood pressure and are on low sodium intake diets, or for the elderly.

▶▶▶ ANTINAUSEANTS

There are at least five different basic causes of nausea. These are: nausea induced by an internal disease, nausea of pregnancy, nausea from motion, nausea from irritation of the stomach, and nausea due to mental upset. Often more than one of these causes will be present simultaneously. Generally, mental upset is present in all forms of nausea and is a strong contributor to the feeling of illness. Most of the things that happen in your stomach are strongly influenced by what's happening in your head.

The type of drug that you should use to aid in nausea depends, to a large degree, on the cause of the nausea. For example, a drug that is useful in the prevention of the nausea of pregnancy is not necessarily useful in nausea induced by motion. It's important to realize that when a drug works to aid in the reduction of nausea or vomiting in one condition it does not mean it will work in a different situation.

Antinauseant drugs are classified by the parts of the body they affect. First, there are those that aid in reducing nausea by coating the stomach and by absorbing or neutralizing irritating materials in the stomach. Drugs of this kind are charcoal, burned toast, antacids, bismuth compounds, and others. Second are drugs that act to relax the muscles of the stomach so as to stop its churning action. These are called "anticholinergic" drugs because the nerves that control the churning of the stomach are "cholinergic" nerves. Drugs of this class are the belladonna derivatives or some synthetic chemicals. I previously discussed some of these, such as scopolamine and a few others. A third group of drugs that will affect the stomach are related to tranquilizers and the antihistamines. These are particularly useful in motion sickness, and are sometimes given for the nausea of pregnancy. Examples are cyclizine, meclizine, dimenhydrinate, chlorpromazine, promethazine, and others. Finally, there are those drugs whose major action is to soothe the mental excitement that contributes to the motion sickness. These are all sedative-hypnotic type drugs, or minor tranquilizers, such as barbiturates, meprobamates, and benzodiazepines.

Coating and Absorbent Drugs

The principal compounds used as gastrointestinal coating and absorbing agents include bismuth subcarbonate, bismuth subnitrate, magnesium trisilicate, aluminum hydroxide, activated charcoal, kaolin, and pectin. Each of these compounds is administered in a dose of between 1 gm and 8 gm over a day to passively absorb any irritating materials that are in the stomach or intestines. Each has its own individual effects in addition to absorbing irritants. Bismuth subcarbonate and bismuth subnitrate give a protective coating to the stomach. Magnesium trisilicate and aluminum hydroxide are antacids. Activated charcoal is one of the most potent of the absorbents but has few other beneficial properties. Kaolin contains aluminum silicate. Therefore, it can also be used for the treatment of diarrhea. The aluminum causes constipation. Pectin is a carbohydrate made by the extraction of the chemical from the rinds of the citrus fruit or apples. It is also useful in the treatment of diarrhea. Kaolin and pectin are usually used together in a mixture of kaolin 20 percent and pectin 1 percent (Kaopectate). Pectin itself is not actually an absorbent. The usual dose of this mixture is 30 ml of solution. These types of antinauseant drugs will be of use only if the nausea is caused by materials in the stomach that are irritating. They are of little or no use for nausea from any other cause.

Anticholinergic Drugs

Drugs that have their effect by stopping stomach churning act by blocking cholinergic nerves. These drugs include atropine, homatropine, atropine methylnitrate, scopolamine, scopolamine hydrobromide (Donphen, Sidonna), homatropine methylbromide, methantheline bromide (Banthine Bromide), propantheline (Pro-Banthine Bromide), oxyphenonium (Antrenyl), anisotropine (Valpin), diphemanil (Prantal), glycopyrrolate (Robinul), hexocyclium (Tral), isopropamide (Darbid), mepenzolate (Cantil), pipenzolate (Piptal), poldine (Nacton), tridihexethyl (Pathilon, Milpath), cyclandelate (Cyclospasmol), eucatropine (Euphthalmine), oxyphencyclimine (Daricon, Vio-thene), piperidolate (Dactil), clidinium (in Librax), and thiphenamil (Trocinate). Two drugs that are general smooth muscle relaxants that affect the muscles of the stomach wall are adiphenine (Trasentine) and dicyclomine (Bentyl). They are different in their means of action from the anticholinergic drugs but end up with the same effect on your stomach. The dose of all the above drugs varies from 1 mg to 40 mg depending on the particular one used. All these drugs act to slow down the nerves that affect the stomach. They are useful in almost all conditions in which a churning action of the stomach is not wanted. Therefore, they are useful for motion sickness, irritation of the stomach, excitement nausea, and in nausea from pregnancy or disease.

Adverse Effects of Anticholinergic Drugs

The problem with all of these anticholinergic drugs is that at an effective dose the side effects are so great that few people will tolerate them. Unfortunately, their effects on the stomach require high doses. Considering atropine as an example of this type of drug, the following are the relative effects of oral doses: at 0.5 mg there is a small degree of slowing of the heart, some dryness of the mouth, and an inhibition of sweating; at 1 mg there is definite dryness of the mouth, some acceleration of heart rate, and mild widening of the eye pupils; at 2 mg there is a rapid heart rate, palpitation of the heart, a marked drying of the mouth, dilation of pupils, and some blurring of vision of near objects. At this dose, you first begin to get an effective slowing of stomach action, with all these other, unpleasant side effects. Few people seem ready to tolerate the extreme dryness of the mouth, rapid heart rate, etc., that accompany a dose that will have any effective action on the stomach. For these reasons, at the recommended dose, most nonprescription antinauseant drugs cause few side effects but are also relatively ineffective in quieting your stomach.

Atropine poisoning can occur at doses between 68 mg and 273 mg. Therefore, the therapeutic safety ratio is about 1:50. Further, its inhibition of sweating can be quite dangerous if you must work hard in a hot climate. Sweating is the predominant means by which the body cools itself. If you cannot sweat and do try to work in a hot environment you are exposing yourself to the risk of heatstroke.

Fortunately, some of the drugs of this type, though they have similar mechanisms of action, have a relatively greater effect upon the stomach than they do upon other parts of your body. One example, methantheline is effective at a dose of 50 mg as an oral tablet in stopping the churning of your stomach. It causes only a small increase in heart rate, inhibition of sweating, blurred vision, or dry mouth at this dose. Scopolamine is somewhat like methantheline. It could be said to lie somewhere between methantheline and atropine in its relative effectiveness without side effects. The dose of scopolamine is lower than either atropine or methantheline. Its usual dose by the oral route is approximately 0.6 mg. However, you should not think that merely because a drug has a greater relative effect on the stomach that you get off scot-free from side effects. Scopolamine causes sedation as well as the other usual side effects of the anticholinergic drugs. The duration of action of anticholinergic-type antinauseants is four to six hours.

Antihistamine-type Antinauseants

Some antihistamines have been found to be rather specific in their effects on an upset stomach due to motion. These antihistamine-type drugs do not have some of the unpleasant side effects of the anticholinergic drugs. These are dimenhydrinate (Dramamine), which is effective at a dose of 50 mg for four to six hours, cyclizine hydrochloride (Marezine), effective at a dose of 50 mg for four to six hours and meclizine hydrochloride (Bonine), at a dose of 25 mg is effective for twelve to twenty-four hours. These are ceiling dose-levels. There is no additional antinauseant effect if taken in greater amounts. Further, although they do not have the unpleasant side effects of the anticholinergic drugs, they have some of their own. They can make you quite drowsy and dizzy. It is an unpleasant form of drowsiness. You feel dragged out. Their effect on motion sickness is obtained only if they are taken at least thirty minutes before the beginning of the motion that will cause you to get sick.

This causes a problem, since you don't always know when you're going to get sick from motion. However, if I were going to go out in a small boat on rough water tomorrow, I would take one of these antihistaminic-type antinauseants thirty to forty-five minutes before going and put up with a drowsy feeling rather than have motion sickness. You have to make your own choice, though, between drug side effects and possible nausea, if you are affected by motion sickness.

Trimethobenzamide (Tigan) is an antinauseant that doesn't quite fit the usual drug classes. It exerts its action directly on the trigger zone for vomiting. At an oral dose of 250 mg, three times a day, it reduces vomiting. It causes drowsiness and can cause tremor or allergic reactions.

Tranquilizer Antinauseants

The final class of antinauseant drugs are tranquilizers. These are chlorpromazine (Thorazine), promethazine (Allergan, Phenergan, Mepergan), meprobamate (Miltown, Equanil); occasionally sedatives of the barbiturate type are used. Promethazine and chlorpromazine are specific antinauseants for the nausea of pregnancy or disease. Chlorpromazine is generally administered between 10 mg and 20 mg orally at one to three times a day. Promethazine is administered between 25 mg and 50 mg orally one to three times a day. Sometimes these are administered either rectally or intramuscularly when vomiting prevents oral administration. This points to the problem that the administration of any drug by the oral route is difficult when nausea and vomiting are present because, even though the pill is vomited, some part of it is absorbed, and it is not known how much was absorbed. This is something to remember. If a pill is taken and then the person vomits, he has had an unknown part of the dose of the drug. It can be dangerous to give him a second pill, for fear he might have absorbed quite a bit of the first pill. If he had, you would be doubling his dose. Chlorpromazine and promethazine are not like the antihistamines in that greater effects accrue with larger doses. They are relatively safe compounds having therapeutic safety ratios of about 1:1,000 or more. Side effects are drowsiness of an unpleasant sort. If they are taken for too long a time, at too high a dose they can cause tremor or, more rarely, jaundice, and, even less frequently, changes in some of the parts of the blood. However, these side effects occur at doses generally far in excess of the amount used for nausea and vomiting. The use of these drugs can result in allergic reactions in some individuals.

▶▶▶ LAXATIVES

There are four types of laxatives. These are: (1) stimulant cathartics, such as castor oil, phenolphthalein, bisacodyl (Dulcolax, Bicol), oxyphenisatin acetate (Acetphenolisatin Isocrin), and cascara sagrada, senna, and danthron (Anavac, Dorbane, Modane); (2) saline cathartics, such as magnesium sulfate (Epsom salts), magnesium hydroxide (Milk of Magnesia), magnesium citrate, magnesium oxide, magnesium carbonate, sodium phosphate, sodium sulfate (Glauber's salt), potassium sodium tartrate (Rochelle salt), and potassium phosphate; (3) bulk-forming laxatives, such as methylcellulose, sodium carboxymethylcellulose, psyllium (plantago), tragacanth, and bran; and (4) emollient laxatives, such as dioctyl sodium sulfosuccinate and mineral oil.

Stimulant Cathartics

The stimulant cathartics differ in some of their individual effects but have many properties in common. They act by stimulating the muscles of the gut, by irritating the mucosa that lines the walls of the intestines, or by selective action on the part of the nervous system that controls intestinal smooth muscles. All of them cause intestinal cramps, increased secretion of fluid, and generally, an excessive elimination of fluid. This is why they cause loose stools and is one of the problems of this type of laxative. Normally, water is picked up in your lower gut from fecal material by reabsorption back into your blood. With cathartics, this water is lost. This can be a serious problem for a person who is already in a state of dehydration because of vomiting or other reasons.

The intensity of cathartic effects is generally proportional to the dose of the stimulant cathartic. These drugs are absorbed into the bloodstream from the gut in differing degrees, but mostly their major effects occur directly inside the intestine. The time of onset of action varies from fast, as with castor oil, which works within three hours, to slow, as with bisacodyl, which starts to work in about six hours.

All laxatives, but particularly the cathartic type, can be dangerous when they are administered to someone who has a stomachache, nausea, vomiting, or cramping. These symptoms might indicate appendicitis. In this disorder, the appendix is already engorged with fecal material and may be in danger of rupturing. The action of a cathartic increases the amount of gut churning, which can force further amounts of fecal material into the appendix and cause it to burst. This is why laxatives, in general, and particularly cathartics, should not be taken by people having gut cramps or aches. You can endanger your life by causing a ruptured appendix.

Saline Laxatives

Saline laxatives include a number of magnesium salts, usually sulfates or tartrates. Mineral waters contain these salts. They act by causing water to be retained in the intestines. This retention of water in the intestine leads to a stimulation of the intestinal muscles, which forces the fecal material out. In this case, as with the stimulant cathartics, the fecal material is semi-fluid and watery. The most common of these laxatives is magnesium sulfate (Epsom salts). Magnesium sulfate is effective in a dose as low as 2 gm to 5 gm, but the usual dose is 15 gm. It produces bowel movement in three to six hours. Milk of magnesia is another of the saline laxatives. It is a mixture of 7 to 9 percent magnesium hydroxide with water. The usual dose is 15 ml of this mixture. It is less effective than 5 gm of magnesium sulfate. Also, it is slower in its time of onset. Other saline laxatives are magnesium oxide, usual dose 4 gm, magnesium carbonate, used at a dose of 8 gm; and magnesium citrate, which has the advantage of being pleasant to taste but more expensive than the others. Sometimes an excess of citric acid and sodium bicarbonate is added to magnesium citrate solution to make it bubble. Its usual dose is 200 ml when in this form.

Some sodium and potassium salts fall within the class of saline laxatives, such as sodium phosphate, sodium sulfate (Glauber's salt), potassium sodium tartrate (Rochelle salt), and potassium phosphate. These sodium salts are similar in their effects to the magnesium salts. Their usual dose is 10 gm. Potassium phosphate, in a dose of 4 gm, has the same general effect. Finally, mineral waters are natural products that contain one or more of the above-mentioned salts. Therefore, they act as saline cathartic laxatives.

The problems caused by saline laxatives are similar to those of stimulant laxatives. They cause activity of the intestinal muscles. This can produce a rupture of the appendix in some cases. Also, these salts are absorbed into the blood to some degree. Persons who chronically use laxatives can get elevated blood levels of the salts. This can cause assorted medical problems. Finally, as with the stimulant laxatives, a water loss is incurred with saline laxatives that can be dangerous if a person is in a dehydrated state.

Bulk-forming Laxatives

Bulk-forming laxatives act by a different means from stimulant or saline laxatives. They do not cause a direct stimulating effect on the muscles of the intestines. They act by dissolving and swelling in the water in the gut to form a lubricating gel or a viscous solution that serves to keep the fecal material soft and wet.

Bulk-forming laxatives are either natural or semi-synthetic derivatives of sugar or cellulose, for example, methylcellulose, sodium carboxymethylcellulose, psyllium (plantago), tragacanth, and bran. They can, by their sheer bulk, aid in producing a bowel movement, but their predominant activity is not so much in causing the bowel movement as in making the bowel movement easier by softening the fecal material and lubricating it. Generally, they do not act until twelve to twenty-four hours after administration. They may take up to three days to act.

The major use of this type of laxative is for people who have hernias, high blood pressure, problems with their stomachs, or heart trouble. These people should not strain while passing fecal material. Thus, to make the bowel movement easier so the person does not have to strain or have the pain of passing hard fecal material over the inflammation of a hernia, he softens and lubricates the fecal matter with a bulk-forming laxative.

These compounds are essentially without direct physiologic action. Therefore, they have very few adverse side effects. Occasionally there has been a case of a person who tried to swallow the dry powders and blocked his throat with them. The only major danger then is in trying to swallow the material itself.

Emollient Laxatives

Emollient laxatives differ from stimulant or saline cathartics. They are similar to bulk-forming laxatives. They do not directly stimulate the gut. Rather, they have the ability to soften and lubricate the fecal matter to make the bowel movement less painful and less stressful.

There are two major types of emollient laxatives: surface-acting agents, and mineral oil. The most common of the surface-acting agents is dioctyl sodium sulfosuccinate (Colace, Doxinate); there are many others. This drug has gained great popularity lately since people have found out that mineral oil has many adverse effects associated with its use. The surface-acting agents soften the fecal materials within twenty-four to forty-eight hours by making the surface of fecal material more permeable to water. They lower the surface tension of the fecal material just like a detergent lowers the surface tension of greases on a dirty frying pan. This action allows the water to penetrate better. This makes the fecal material soft and wet.

The recommended oral doses of dioctyl sodium sulfosuccinate can be as large as 50 mg/kg even in infants. It has not been shown to have adverse effects. However, in animals very large doses of the drug have produced vomiting and diarrhea. It comes in 50-mg or 100-mg tablets or capsules for oral administration, or as a syrup, with 4 mg per ml or about 50 mg per tablespoon. The recommended dose varies, but is usually between 50 mg and 200 mg daily for an adult. For children of less than three years of age, the dose is as low as 10 mg to 40 mg. Another surface-acting agent is poloxyalkol (Magsol, Polykol). It is similar to dioctyl sodium sulfosuccinate in its activities. It is available for oral administration in 250 mg tablets and solutions of 50 mg to 250 mg per ml. The recommended dose for children under three years of age is 100 mg to 200 mg once or twice daily, older children 200 mg one to three times daily, and adults 200 mg two to four times daily.

Mineral oil is the classic drug used to soften fecal material to make its passage easier. It is the oil itself that softens the fecal matter to make it slide better. Mineral oil can cause a variety of adverse effects. Few people seem to appreciate its potential hazards to health. With better, safer drugs now available, I wonder why it is used at all. Habitual use is clearly to be avoided. Mineral oil can be inspired into the lungs. When it gains access to the lungs a disorder called fat pneumonia can develop. This is particularly hazardous in debilitated or elderly individuals. Further, mineral oil blocks the absorption of vitamins A and D. Finally, mineral oil can leak past the muscles in the anus to cause the rather annoying side effect of itching. All in all, it is difficult to understand why people would use something with the potential dangers of mineral oil. Its use, even as a low calorie salad oil, should be avoided.

There are a number of laxatives that have become outmoded because of their danger. However, you can still occasionally find them in some traditional medicines. One example of these obsolete laxatives is calomel, which is mercury chloride. Although this was once one of the most popular of all laxatives, its use is almost completely gone because of the possibility of mercury poisoning. Aloe is another that has been given up because it causes tremendous irritation in the lower gut and pelvic regions. Pills of aloe, strychnine, and belladonna (ASB pills) were once frequently given to children. These sometimes caused strychnine poisoning. Also, a number of resins have been used in the past as laxatives. Now they have been discarded since they caused considerable irritation of the gut and watery stools. They could lead to dehydration and death when used in too great an amount. These are jalap, colocynth, elaterin, ipomoea, gamboge, and podophyllum.

Dependence on Laxatives

You should know that a true dependence can be developed by the chronic use of laxatives, and many gastrointestinal disturbances in adults can be traced to the habitual use of laxative substances. Therefore, if you have continued constipation, it would seem the wisest course to go to a physician to find out its cause, rather than taking laxatives, on a continuing basis, because you have a belief that you should be completely "regular."

▶▶▶ ANTIDIARRHEALS

Diarrhea can be caused by many diseases. However, the most common causes are an irritable gut that is too active or taking an antibiotic that kills all the intestinal germs that help the body process food on its way through. This effect of antibiotics is discussed in more detail in the chapter on antibiotics.

There are three kinds of antidiarrheal drugs, which are used alone or in combination. One type helps to absorb excess water in order to thicken the fecal material, such as kaolin or one of the bulk-forming laxatives. The second kind are the anticholinergic drugs mentioned in the section on antacids, such as scopolamine or atropine. These drugs slow the excess gut activity. Finally, the most effective antidiarrheals are derivatives of opium, such as paregoric or diphenoxylate (Lomotil). These drugs will be discussed in more detail in the chapter on analgesics. They can literally stop all gut movement.

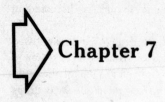

Chapter 7

Analgesics

Analgesics are drugs that are used to relieve pain. At one time or another in our lives all of us have pain and seek relief from it by the use of drugs. Indeed, analgesics are the most often purchased drugs in the United States. It seems that we hurt a lot.

▶▶▶ THE NATURE OF PAIN

To understand the way analgesics act to reduce pain, you must understand something about pain itself. When your body hurts, it is trying to tell you something. Your body normally is not supposed to have continuous or severe pain. Therefore, when you have a severe or continuing pain you should wonder what is causing the pain. If your first impulse is to rush to take a drug that will reduce your suffering, without considering what the cause of the pain is, you may be turning a deaf ear to something important that your body is trying to tell you. A friend of mine once proposed that the solution to the population problem, and to the drug problem, was to make all pain-relieving drugs easily available without prescription. Then when intelligent, sensible people had pain, they would go to see a physician to find out what caused it. The unintelligent, unwise people would not find the cause of the pain but would just take a drug to relieve it. They would not cure the problem. In a short while, these foolish people, who ignored the warnings of their body, would die. This would solve both the population and the drug problems at once. Although my friend was joking at the time, I must admit there was some element of sense in his proposal. The moral to this proposal is not that you shouldn't use pain-relieving drugs. If you have a constant or severe pain and have established the cause of the pain, then the pain is no longer serving any useful function for you. I have seen few, if any, people whose personality or character was improved by suffering.

Notice that I have been talking about constant or severe pain. I've used these terms because there is an average pain level for all people. If you attend to yourself very closely, you will soon notice that, at a rate of about twenty times an hour, you will have mild twinges here or there in your head, body, muscles, and so on. This is the normal level of discomfort to which all of us have to adjust. It does not indicate anything particular is wrong with you. Usually these small pains cause relatively little suffering unless you dwell upon the feelings and start to worry about them. Probably, the best way to handle such average pain is to just ignore it.

True pathologic pain is caused by heat, pressure, or body chemicals that stimulate special pain nerves in your body. Pain relief comes from either causing your brain to be inattentive to the signals of these special nerves or by directly blocking the effects of heat, pressure, or chemicals on the pain nerves. When I speak of heat, pressure, or chemicals I mean not only these stressors from the outside, but also the heat, pressure, or chemicals that are produced within your own body in response to disease, infection, irritation, or wounding.

105 ◀◀◀

▶▶ PHYSICAL METHODS FOR PAIN RELIEF

There are a number of physical methods that will relieve certain kinds of pain. For example, if you have a headache caused by high blood pressure in the arteries on the outside layer of your temples, a common method of relieving this pain is to put pressure on the sides of the bridge of your nose. This pressure will reduce the flow of blood to the blood vessels on the sides of your head. Similarly, mountain climbers who are climbing at very high altitudes, ten thousand feet or more, often get headaches because of the reduced amount of oxygen in their environment. This headache can often be relieved by a tight headband, which reduces the pressure of the blood in the superficial arteries of the head. Another physical method for pain relief that is effective for sore, stiff muscles is heat — particularly hot, moist packs. The usual reason that muscles hurt after exercise or from tension is that part of the muscle is in a sustained contraction. This contraction can reduce the amount of blood getting to the muscle. The muscle cells react to this lack of blood flow, with a concomitant lack of an adequate oxygen supply to the muscle, by the release of minute amounts of chemicals called kinins. These act directly upon the special nerves that cause pain. Heat, or sometimes mild exercise, will cause an increased blood flow to these suffocating, suffering muscles. This relieves the condition of low oxygen that stops the release of the kinins, thus doing away with the pain. Whether or not to exercise a muscle to relieve cramping and pain is in some dispute. There seems to be three schools of thought. One group believes that exercise helps. A second group believes that stretching the muscles will relieve the pain. Finally, a third belief is that immobilization of the muscle plus hot packs is best. I've heard many and varied arguments as to which of these is the best approach. I have no particularly strong opinion myself, since for me sometimes one method works and sometimes another. I suppose if I were forced into having to make a choice of which technique seems to work most often for me, I would choose hot packs and immobilization. But I wouldn't bet a lot on that choice over other possibilities.

▶▶ THE PSYCHOLOGICAL RELIEF OF PAIN

There also are psychological methods for the relief of pain. The first, and perhaps preferable, method is to ignore the pain. If pain is at a low level and can be ignored, this is probably the best approach. Many times it is not the pain itself that causes the suffering so much as excessive worry about the pain. If you can ignore the pain, not worry about it, you're probably better off. Another pain-relief approach is distraction. If you can become very interested in something else, it will help you forget the fact that you hurt. This only works if the pain is moderate or low level. Finally, there is belief. By believing that you feel better, a great deal of the suffering of pain can be relieved. This has been shown in many experiments. Inactive drugs, or a drug at a very low dose, called "placebos" are often very effective in relieving pain if the person receiving them thinks they are an active, pain-relieving drug. As you will recall from the previous chapter, a "placebo" effect occurs when either a fake drug is given or a drug is given at a dose that is below its threshold of action but still produces an improvement because the person expects it to. Even when the placebo effect is tested in hospitals by giving postoperative patients injections of plain water, about 30 to 50 percent of the patients, believing they have received a pain-reducing drug, will experience a marked reduction in degree of pain. This demonstrates how strongly belief and attitude can intensify or reduce the suffering from pain.

▶▶ PAIN RELIEF BY DRUGS

Drugs that relieve pain either work directly at the site of the pain itself or work on the pain interpretation center in the brain. Common drugs that work at the site of pain itself are counterirritants, mild analgesics, surface anesthetics, and muscle relaxants. Drugs that alter the interpretation of pain in the brain are the potent analgesics. A few special drugs that are not true analgesics but can reduce the pain in particular conditions such as gout, arthritis, and migraine, will also be discussed.

Mild Analgesics

Aspirin

Of all analgesics, aspirin is the most used and useful drug in the world. Literally tons upon tons of aspirin (acetylsalicylic acid) is used either alone or in combination with other drugs. Yet, historically aspirin is a relatively new drug. It came into use in the late 1800s. However, it was such an effective drug that its use quickly spread all over the world.

Aspirin works at the site of the pain by three actions. First, it reduces the swelling that occurs at a site of injury or infection. This, in turn, reduces the pressure on the pain nerves. Second, it reduces the heat generated by the flow of blood and inflammation at a site of injury or infection. Third, it directly blocks the pain-causing chemicals, the kinins, that are released at a site of injury and that act upon the pain nerves. Aspirin also works in the brain. It acts to reduce fever. As you can see from all these different modes of pain relief, aspirin is good for the relief of not only the pain of simple headache but also any type of pain or irritation you might have. It is a vastly underrated drug.

As I mentioned earlier, the threshold dose of aspirin is about 300 mg (5 gr) and its ceiling dose for the reduction of simple pain occurs at 900 mg (15 gr). Its time-action is about four hours. Aspirin is readily absorbed from the stomach in whatever form you take it. Its onset time varies from ten to forty-five minutes, depending upon what else is in your stomach and the form of the aspirin. Aspirin combined with sodium bicarbonate or some other buffering substance or carbonated aspirin (aspirin that fizzes), tends to be absorbed fastest. However, aspirin dissolved in hot water is just as fast. Aspirin, just as a standard pill, is still readily and easily absorbed almost as quickly.

Adverse Effects of Aspirin. Aspirin is not without its hazards. First, you should appreciate that an acute overdose of aspirin is the single biggest cause of death by drugs in young children in the United States. About one hundred sixty-five to two hundred people die each year from aspirin overdose in our country. The lethal dose of aspirin in an adult is between 10 gm and 30 gm. In children as low as 5 gm (17 to 20 regular 300-mg aspirin tablets) can be lethal. Second, a few people are allergic to aspirin. This allergy can manifest itself in a number of ways. An extremely rare form of response is death within a few minutes of taking one or two aspirin. The allergic mechanism of the body puts the person into shock. The lowered blood pressure of the shock causes death. Fortunately, this is a very rare reaction, but it has occurred. A greater number of people have a mild allergic response to aspirin. This is the itch, flare, and wheal caused by histamine release. Third, aspirin, though it is a very mild acid, is generally contraindicated in patients who have peptic ulcers. Even as mild an acid as aspirin can further irritate the stomach. The same would be true for any person who had any form of stomach inflammation. Indeed, in a healthy person taking aspirin, a small amount of blood is released in the stomach due to its irritating effect. However, the amount of blood released is less than a teaspoonful. For example, if you took three standard aspirin tablets four times a day you might lose 5 ml of blood. This causes no particular damage to a normal stomach. After all, you have 5 liters of blood in your body. You can easily spare one teaspoonful without any problem. Finally, there is the problem of chronic aspirin use. Aspirin reduces the ability of your blood to clot. This is not so severe an effect that it will cause you to bleed to death, but people who chronically use aspirin do tend to have bruises all over. The small blood vessels that are broken in a bruise are not as readily repaired in chronic, excessive aspirin users. You can almost always tell a chronic, excessive aspirin user. He will be black and blue all over. On the whole, however, aspirin is a useful and effective pain-relieving drug. Its effectiveness is often underrated since it is so common. It's really very good.

The precise form of the aspirin has to be taken into account. About 5 percent of all people who take aspirin may get an upset stomach. This occurs most often in people who take aspirin on an empty stomach or who take a type of aspirin that breaks up in the stomach into relatively large pieces. If aspirin is taken with milk or is of a type that breaks into very small particles, the incidence of upset stomach is somewhat less than the usual 5 percent. Much ado has been made in advertising about gastric upset caused by aspirin. Consider that this occurs in only about 5 percent of the population and the odds are one in twenty that you will be a person who gets a stomach upset with aspirin. If you wish to pay the price of aspirin combined with buffering products, such as sodium bicarbonate, or a very fine particulate aspirin for more adequate dispersal in your stomach, you can. On the other hand, you can coat your stomach by taking aspirin with a little milk (although that slows the absorption of the aspirin somewhat). It will protect you from any mild irritation. Then you can use a cheaper brand of aspirin. I do.

Acetaminophen

Another type of drug used alone or in combination with aspirin is phenacetin (Acetophenetidin) or acetaminophen (Arthralgen, Febrogesic, Datril, Tempra, Tylenol, and many others). Phenacetin, which is the P of APC, is a fairly common drug. Phenacetin and acetaminophen are really the same drug. Phenacetin is converted into acetaminophen in the body before it becomes active. The usual oral dose of either phenacetin or acetaminophen is between 300 mg and 600 mg for adults and older children, 100 mg for young children. Its onset time is similar to that of aspirin as is its time-action of three to four hours. These drugs are analgesics of the same type as aspirin. They can also cause reduction in fever. However, they do not act to reduce swelling nor do they reduce the heat at sites of inflammation. For this reason they are less effective as drugs for rheumatic disorders, blisters, or muscle pain. These drugs can be substituted for aspirin for people who are allergic to aspirin. They are no more effective than aspirin nor do they add to aspirin's effectiveness beyond its ceiling dose of 900 mg.

There are hazards associated with the use of phenacetin and acetaminophen. They can cause a particular form of anemia that can affect about 10 percent of Negroes. The condition is relatively rare among Caucasians. However, all people can have damage to the kidney if large doses of these two drugs are taken, or even at the usual therapeutic doses if they are taken regularly for over ten days. Acetaminophen causes fewer adverse effects than phenacetin. All in all, it seems that these drugs have little advantage over aspirin for the treatment of pain except for those people who are allergic to aspirin. Indeed, for some types of pain due to swelling and inflammation they are inferior to aspirin.

Commonly, you will find combinations with drugs of the phenacetin type added to aspirin, possibly with caffeine also. APCs are aspirin, phenacetin, and caffeine. There is little evidence that shows that the addition of a phenacetin to aspirin adds to its ability to relieve pain. The addition of caffeine to the mixture does not contribute to pain reduction unless the pain is due specifically to a headache caused by high blood pressure in the blood vessels in your head. One cup of coffee or a cola can give you an equivalent amount if you want it. This seems to me to be a cheaper and pleasanter way to get caffeine.

My own approach to the use of the analgesics for moderate pain is to buy the cheapest aspirin I can find on sale, as long as it has the initial "USP" behind it. I look for those initials because they stand for "United States Pharmacopeia." This ensures that there has been an adequate control of the purities of the aspirin. Next, I know that when aspirin is exposed to air, it picks up water. When it picks up water, it loses potency. To overcome this loss of effectiveness I take

111 ◀◀◀

three aspirin instead of two. I do not expect miracles of speed. I wait for at least forty-five minutes before I expect the pain to go away. Also, I do not take more aspirin or any other kind of mild analgesic for at least four hours since I have taken the ceiling dose. Finally, if pain persists beyond a day or becomes quite severe, I forget about trying to treat myself and scurry to a physician so he can look for the cause of the pain.

Surface Analgesics and Anesthetics

Some types of pain-relieving drugs are used by rubbing them into the skin over the site of pain, by taking them as throat lozenges or gargles onto irritated membranes of the throat and mouth, or by inserting as a suppository in the rectum. These analgesics are of two types: first, counterirritants and second, local anesthetics.

Counterirritants

Counterirritants are substances that when spread upon the skin will cause an expansion of local blood vessels that increases blood flow. They produce a degree of irritation and warming. They act by two means. First, when they're used on sore, stiff muscles, they increase the blood flow, not only locally to the skin to which they are applied but also to the underlying muscles. This increased blood flow to the muscles does not occur because of the drug penetrating into the muscles but because of the way the body's nerves are arranged in skin and muscle. When there is a high rate of blood flow to your skin, blood also automatically flows into the muscle under the skin. If the cause of your muscle pain is due to a lack of adequate oxygen in your muscle caused by a constriction of your blood vessels, then increasing blood flow to the muscle will provide it with more oxygen. This will cause the pain to be relieved.

Counterirritant analgesics also act by confusing the pain nerves.

These drugs produce a mild warming and irritation of the skin. This masks pain nerve activity. You might think of the effect as similar to trying to hear a specific person's screeching voice while a loud band is playing. The band noise masks the person's voice. In the same way, the mild irritation of the analgesic masks the pain nerves' specific signals to your brain.

The major constituents of counterirritant analgesics are irritant oils. For example, menthol is an oil obtained from peppermint oil, which stimulates nerves to feel a perception of cold but which depresses pain nerves. It is usually found in a concentration of from 0.25 to 1.0 percent in most commonly used counterirritants. It is effective for this purpose but can be dangerous or lethal if accidentally swallowed. Methyl salicylate is another counterirritant that can also be dangerous. Any mixture containing over 5 percent methyl salicylate must carry a warning label. It acts upon the skin causing the sensation of either cooling or warming. It is quite often considered too strong to be placed among the usual liniments or lotions. Cinnamon oil is a strong irritant in very low concentrations. It also will be found among the counterirritants beside these other oils. Chloroform is often used in counterirritants not because it has any great strength as a counterirritant but because it helps mix the other chemicals, though it does have some irritant properties. Oil of mustard is occasionally used, sometimes indicated by its chemical name of alioisothycyanate. However, generally speaking, it is considered too strong an irritant for topical application, particularly if there is to be any type of bandage covering. Indeed, any of the liniments when covered can produce second degree burns on the body. This is like a very bad sunburn. Capsicum oleoresin can produce a great warmth on the body, yet very little redness. The mechanism by which this occurs is not known. Finally, methacholine chloride and histamine dihydrochloride at concentrations varying between 0.1 and 1.0 percent are employed, though these are not irritant oils, because they produce a local dilation of the blood vessels by another mechanism. Besides the compounds I've mentioned, various other chemicals can be used.

Generally, counterirritants are carried in a greaseless base, lanolin base, soap, alcohol, rosemary or pine oil, glycerin, or kerosene. Some of these bases also have some irritant properties. For the most part they serve primarily as carriers or vehicles for the other substances. Frankly, the various commercial counterirritants all seem to be about the same to me. The only basis for choosing one over another would be its strength, that is, whether it warms you without discomfort, the type of base it is in, and the odor you might prefer. Actually hot, wet packs will probably work as well or better to relieve your pain.

Local Anesthetics

The local anesthetics directly stop pain by interfering with the transmission of signals by special pain nerves. These substances are derivatives of cocaine. Most of us have had experience with some of these drugs in the dental chair, in the form of novocaine or xylocaine (Lidocaine), in throat lozenges and gargles as benzocaine, or in ointments as dibucaine. Cocaine, as well as its various derivatives, is a potent, effective anesthetic agent that will stop local pain. When rubbed onto the skin it is partially absorbed. This gives even a deeper pain relief.

Often you will find these drugs given by injection into or just under a specific area of the skin. This eliminates the pain that might be caused when a dentist is drilling a tooth or that comes when pulling a tooth, or when a physician wishes to do a minor surgical procedure such as sewing up a small wound. These drugs are effective, and there is little danger associated with their usual use. The only problem that can occur in such injections is by accident. If the drug is accidentally injected into an artery or vein it can get into your bloodstream. These drugs are potent blockers of the heart. If a small amount is injected directly into your circulatory system it can cause your heart to stop for a moment. You would experience this as a sudden dizziness and nausea and, possibly, a momentary loss of consciousness. Luckily this is a rare event. The mistake is seldom made. To ensure that he is not directly injecting into a vein or an artery, your physician or dentist as a common practice will pull the plunger on his syringe out a little after he has made the insertion with the needle. In this way he can ensure that there is no blood in the syringe, as there would have been if he had hit a vein or an artery. The effectiveness of these drugs in slowing or stopping the heart is used, occasionally, in emergency procedures when the heart is out of control and it is imperative to slow the heart down as a lifesaving measure. However, this is an extremely dangerous procedure. It is only used when a physician is sure that it is absolutely necessary to save a life.

Benzocaine is a derivative of cocaine that is not absorbed into the blood through the membranes of either the mouth or the throat, or through the skin. Therefore, it is both safe and effective in deadening the superficial pain nerves in these areas. This is why lotions, sprays, ointments, or lozenges containing between 5 and 20 percent benzocaine are often used for sore throats, sunburn, and other conditions where there is surface irritation. A problem can occur if benzocaine is directly placed on an open wound. Then it can get directly into the bloodstream with possible effects on your heart.

Benzocaine compounds are probably oversold. They are effective, but a cold bath, followed by stroking the irritated area with a cloth bag full of cooked oatmeal to protect the skin, is probably as effective and useful an analgesic for irritation as any of the commercial preparations containing benzocaine. A cold bath takes away most of the pain and the oatmeal coats the skin so that there is no further irritation. The old idea of butter for irritation or burns is incorrect. Also, soaking an extensive burned area in tea is dangerous. The tannin in the tea can cause tannic acid poisoning.

Very often the commercial medications containing local anesthetics for irritation or sunburn also contain various antiseptics, such as benzalkonium chloride or hexachlorophene. At this time, there is little evidence that any of these extra ingredients do any good for you at all. The correct treatment of infection is with antibiotics taken internally, not antiseptics applied externally. Anyway, it is very unlikely you would have an infection in the above-mentioned cases. Further, some of these chemicals, such as hexachlorophene, can easily penetrate burned tissue. You can get a rather high level of hexachlorophene in your blood from such an application. Therefore, it's probably more dangerous than useful to have these added antiseptics.

Potent Analgesics

The derivatives of the opium poppy have perhaps been the most beneficial to mankind over the years of any single type of drug. Also, these same derivatives of the opium poppy have probably been the subject of more misinformation and unnecessary fear than any other single type of drug. It's interesting to observe the confusion that has built up around these drugs. For indeed, their use goes back to ancient times. They have been very well studied for many years, yet all sorts of irrational ideas exist about them.

The History of Opium

As I mentioned before, as early as 1000 B.C., the Egyptians used the extract of the opium poppy, opium, to induce sleep and eliminate pain. All through the Middle Ages, particularly in Arabic medicine, opium was understood to relieve the suffering of pain. As early as the twelfth century Arab physicians recognized that if one took too much opium, consistently day after day, for too long a time, a physical dependence could develop. Our own experience with physical dependence on the derivatives of opium first developed during the Civil War. Morphine, the active principle of opium, had been extracted from raw opium gum. It was given by hypodermic to wounded soldiers in pain. Since Western countries did not understand the nature of physical dependence at this time, many of the soldiers developed a dependence on morphine. Morphine dependence was called "the soldier's disease." At about this time, heroin (diacetyl morphine) was introduced into American medicine. It was believed that heroin did not produce physical dependence. They certainly were wrong.

Much of the mythology that surrounds opium, morphine, and heroin use grew up with the building of the western railroads. Chinese were imported into the western United States to lay the track. They brought with them the habit of smoking opium. It is during this era that the image of the opium den as a place of crime and terror developed. In actuality, an opium den is not a place of crime and terror but rather a very tranquil place, a place for sleep and relaxation. Another mistaken impression developed at this point was the idea that the Chinese were the developers and major users of opium. This is not true. Opium was brought to China by the British from the Middle East. For years this was one of the big money makers for British trading. The British Opium Wars were fought against China when the empress of China tried to block the trade in opium to keep her people from being exploited by the British. China was the first country in relatively modern times to have laws regulating the use and supply of opium. In China, at the time of the Opium Wars, the death penalty was prescribed for the use of opium. However, since the British had greater force of arms, the empress of China's resolve to keep her country free of opiates was broken and the British continued to bring in opium. Then, at a later date, the Chinese brought the habit into the United States.

The Actions of Opiates

Since the original use of raw opium for medicine, literally thousands of different derivatives of opium and synthetic opiates have been prepared. Most of these are relatively uncommon so, for the purposes of this book, I will discuss only the following common opiates: paregoric (tincture of brown opium), morphine, codeine (monomethylmorphine), methadone, oxycodone (Percodan), heroin (diacetylmorphine), and meperidine (Demerol).

Morphine is the major chemical that acts in the body regardless of whether the drug that you take is paregoric, codeine, or heroin. They are all converted to morphine in your body. Meperidine is a synthetic opiate but its properties are so similar to those of morphine that it does not deserve separate discussion. Paregoric is an alcohol solution of pure opium. Opium contains about 10 percent morphine. So the active principle of paregoric is morphine. Heroin and morphine are badly absorbed in the stomach. Thus, they must be given by injection. Codeine and oxycodone are absorbed through the stomach relatively easily. They can be given orally. But absorption into the brain from the blood is different. Heroin is fastest, morphine is not as fast, and codeine is slowest in rate of absorption into the brain from the blood. Thus, you could say that heroin is a "fast-acting morphine" and the codeine is a "slow-acting morphine." Meperidine and oxycodone are essentially identical to morphine in rate of absorption into the brain. The time-action of these opiates for pain relief is about three to four hours.

All opiates have three major therapeutic uses. These are: (1) the relief of fear and suffering, (2) the production of constipation to stop diarrhea, and (3) the suppression of coughing. These therapeutic properties of the opiates are directly caused by their actions on the nervous system. The opiates have the adverse effect of slowing the brain center that governs breathing. This is the cause of death when an overdose of an opiate is taken; breathing stops. The opiates cause sweating, constriction of the pupils of the eyes, nausea and vomiting. If a person who is not in pain, who is not suffering, or who is not sick is given any of the opiates without having been told what he is being given (to block any expectations), he will usually report that the drug causes a very unpleasant experience. On the other hand, if an opiate is given to a suffering person, he will experience a pleasant and dramatic relief from his suffering.

The drug methadone (Dolophine, Amidone, Methenex) has received a great deal of attention lately. Methadone is an opiate that has the same actions as morphine, heroin, codeine, meperidine, or oxycodone. It differs only in that it is more slowly absorbed and excreted than the other opiates. It is a bit less potent than morphine and is effective when taken orally. Morphine and heroin have little effect when given by mouth. One may take methadone by mouth once a day and its effects will last for twenty-four hours. The time-action of the other opiates is only four to six hours. It is this long time-action and effectiveness by the oral route that have made methadone useful as a substitute for heroin in opiate dependent people.

The primary use of all the derivatives of opium is to relieve suffering. To make the distinction between pain and suffering, many things can cause suffering, and pain is only one of them. The opiates will reduce suffering regardless of the cause. If you ask a person who is taking an opiate whether he still hurts, he'll say yes, but he won't care as much anymore. This general relief from all types of suffering may be part of the reason that opiates are taken by people who are not in physical pain but who are suffering from mental pain or anguish. How opiates cause this effect in the brain is not known.

Morphine given by injection has a threshold dose for suffering at a level of about 5 mg. The usual maximum dose given therapeutically is 20 mg. The lethal dose of morphine is between five to ten times the therapeutic dose for a person who has not developed tolerance. Codeine, when taken orally, which is its usual form, is effective in the relief of pain at a dose of 32 mg to 60 mg. The lethal dose of codeine is approximately ten to fifteen times the therapeutic dose. Oxycodone is very similar to codeine. It is sometimes given by injection at a dose of 10 mg to 15 mg. It can be given orally. The therapeutic dose range of heroin (diacetylmorphine), in those countries in which it is used therapeutically, is approximately 2.5 mg to 10 mg. It is not used therapeutically in the United States. Since it is absorbed into the brain more readily than pure morphine, it is slightly more potent, perhaps by 50 percent. In the brain, the extra acetyl groups, which make it different from morphine, are split off heroin to turn it into morphine. Heroin is morphine when it acts in the brain. Meperidine is effective therapeutically in an oral dose between 50 mg and 100 mg. As an injection it is used at between 10 mg and 30 mg. For heroin and meperidine, the lethal dose in persons who have developed no tolerance to the drug is approximately five to ten times that used for therapeutic purposes.

Codeine is often combined with other medications, such as aspirin, to produce a pain-relieving pill. Thirty-two mg of codeine is approximately equal in analgesic effectiveness to two or three aspirin. However, when you put aspirin and codeine together you get about twice the analgesic effect, at least, and possibly even more. Aspirin works predominantly at the site of the pain, particularly if it's a pain of inflammation or soreness. The opiates work by a completely different mechanism. They reduce the suffering of the pain, rather than the pain itself. These two types of action then can combine to give greater pain relief than either alone could give.

All the opiates cause a constant contraction of the muscles in the stomach and the intestines. This gives them the ability to cause constipation, since the muscles cannot follow the rhythmic contractions required for bowel movement. Rather, they are held in constant contraction all the time. Historically, this has been one of the greatest uses of opiates — for the treatment of disorders where diarrhea can become life-threatening, such as cholera, dysentery, and so on. In these diseases people die from the dehydration caused by excessive water loss. Anything that will stop the bowel from putting out fluid, so it can be reabsorbed to allow the body to retain water, can be lifesaving.

The third property of the opiates that is used therapeutically is their ability to cause a depression of the cough center so that one can stop coughing. The most common opiates used for this are codeine or dextromethorphan (Romilar). Codeine may be obtained as an elixir, such as elixir terpin hydrate or wild cherry syrup (Cheracol). These syrups contain 32 mg of codeine per 0.5 ounce in an alcohol solution with either terpin hydrate to impart orange flavor, or wild cherry syrup to impart a cherry flavor to an otherwise unpalatable mixture. The usual dose for cough suppression is a teaspoonful when needed, not to exceed 2 ounces a day maximum. Dextromethorphan is similar to codeine as a cough suppressant but has no analgesic or dependence producing properties. Its use is coming to be preferred over codeine because it does not produce dependence. It can be purchased without a prescription.

You can develop tolerance of all the opiates mentioned except dextromethorphan. Tolerance, as I previously described, means that if you take the drug constantly it will take greater and greater amounts of the drug to achieve the same effect. Further, there is a tolerance built up to the lethal properties of the drugs, namely, depression of the respiratory center. Once again, however, the rate at which the tolerance builds to the therapeutic or desired effects is faster than the rate at which tolerance develops to the lethal effects. This causes a number of problems, particularly in the illegal drug market where dosage is so badly controlled. To get the desired effect you get closer and closer to the lethal effect. A person who is highly tolerant of heroin or morphine can take in as much as 300 mg to 500 mg each day with impunity. For this type of person, it may take up to 1,000 mg or more to cause death. However, if a person has a low level of tolerance, perhaps taking in as little as 80 mg of drug in a single dose may kill him.

It is not necessary to develop excessive tolerance or dependence on opiates if the schedule of administration is carefully controlled. By regulation of dose and number of doses per day, one may keep the degree of tolerance from developing to a high level. For this reason, medically caused tolerance of or dependence on opiates is so rare as to be unimportant. If anything, physicians are too conservative, allowing patients to suffer unnecessarily because of a fear of dependence.

Opiate Dependence

The opiates produce both psychological and physiological dependence. Again, by psychological dependence, we mean that some people like the mental state that the drug produces and so tend to seek it. As I mentioned earlier, if you are not suffering when you are first exposed to the opiates, you will not have a pleasurable experience. However, after a person has been taking the drug in an adequate quantity, for a long enough period of time, the desire to regain the drugged state, which has then become pleasurable, is very strong. The drug experience of a dependent person is described as a warm feeling, starting at the pit of the stomach and then spreading out over the rest of the body. It's sort of like floating on a warm, pink cloud. The person then becomes rather sleepy. This state is called the "nods."

It takes longer to develop physical dependence on the opiates than most people realize. In experimental studies, it has been shown that if one takes heroin at a high rate, at ever-increasing doses, all day long, every day, it will still take ten solid days of drug administration at high dose levels before even mild withdrawal symptoms are shown when the heroin is abruptly withdrawn. Since physical dependence is defined by a physiological upset of some degree upon the cessation of the drug, we may say that ten days seems to be about as fast as this dependence can develop. One should note though that this requires the taking of a relatively high dose of the drug five to six times daily to cause this level of physical dependence in ten days. The average person obtaining opiates on the street usually takes a period of months or years to become dependent.

The nature of the withdrawal reaction to the opiates is much misunderstood as a result of a great deal of propaganda in the movies, books, and on TV. Withdrawal from the opiates is characterized by the onset of illness in about twenty-four hours. It peaks at about seventy-two hours and is over in four to five days. The state of the person during this time is characterized by rapid beating of the heart, widening of the pupils, sweating, severe stomach cramps and, of course, a desire for the opiates that will relieve these symptoms. People do not tend to be violent. Indeed, it is very difficult to be very violent when you're having a severe stomach cramp. Those patients I have seen during withdrawal lie on their beds, with their knees up against their chests, because of the stomach cramps, and say, "Doctor, I'm sick." Further, as I mentioned previously, an abrupt withdrawal of the barbiturates or of alcohol causes hallucinations and delusions called delirium tremens (DTs). These are not present in opiate withdrawal. Further, 15 percent can die on abrupt withdrawal of alcohol or barbiturates, only 1 to 3 percent of severely dependent, physically ill people die on abrupt withdrawal of opiates. The difference between an opiate withdrawal and the alcohol or barbiturate DTs is about the same as the difference between a bad case of the flu and something as severe as a heart attack.

Dependence on any drug, whether it is alcohol, opiate, barbiturate, or other, has one characteristic that makes it a frightening phenomenon. This is the relapse rate, that is, going back to its use again and again. We have no adequate treatment for people who have become dependent upon drugs. The majority of people who have become dependent on any drug will usually relapse at least once, probably many more times, before they give up the habit. Once a drug habit has been installed it is very hard to stop. We have yet to find any successful means of truly eliminating the habit to the extent that the person will not go back to drug use at some time or other in their lives.

Much has been said of late about the use of methadone in the detoxification or maintenance of persons who have become dependent upon opiates. Whether you are for this approach or against it, you must consider that methadone is just another opiate. It can cause dependence. It is sort of an oral, long-lasting morphine. Methadone maintenance programs allow the person who has become dependent to obtain the drug that he needs. It prevents him from going into withdrawal. He receives his drug from an approved, medical source as opposed to getting it from a pusher on the street. He receives it at a low cost, as opposed to the very high cost of heroin from the pusher. He gets a reliable drug in quality and dosage as compared to the unknown quality and quantity he gets obtaining drugs on the street. He receives methadone in an oral form, as opposed to intravenous "mainlining" with heroin or morphine. Methadone lasts for twenty-four hours, as opposed to four to six hours for heroin or morphine. No one will contend that methadone is a cure for dependence upon opiates. It is a replacement by one opiate, with potentially more desirable properties from society's viewpoint, for another opiate that has many undesirable properties from society's viewpoint. It is used because we have no effective therapy that will prevent many people from relapsing into drug use once they have developed a very strong habit.

Many people regard paregoric and codeine as benign drugs. This is almost true but not totally so. It is estimated that there are about one thousand people in this country who are physically dependent upon codeine or paregoric. However, these people are usually not the type who use heroin. They do not get picked up by the police, do not cause crimes, and they do not make newspaper headlines. Quite often they are nice little old ladies who go from drugstore to drugstore refilling their codeine cough syrup bottles over and over. It takes a great deal of paregoric or codeine to cause dependence because these drugs are poorly absorbed. But since paregoric is effective because it contains 10 percent morphine, and codeine is monomethylmorphine, which is converted into morphine in the body, these drugs do have a slight potential for physical dependence.

Opiates with a Low Liability for Dependence

There are a series of new opiate-like drugs that differ from the others because they do not cause the same type of dependence as the other opiates. These are diphenoxylate (Lomotil), dextromethorphan, propoxyphene (Darvon), ethoheptazine citrate (Zactirin), and pentazocine (Talwin). Diphenoxylate is a derivative of the same series of opiates as meperidine, but it has a very low potential for the development of dependence. This doesn't mean dependence can't occur, but that it takes a tremendous amount of the drug for a tremendous length of time to get dependence. Diphenoxylate is used predominantly for the treatment of diarrhea. It capitalizes on the constipating properties of the opiate.

Ethoheptazine citrate and propoxyphene are both used as analgesics. Quite often they are used in combination with aspirin, as is codeine. Their potency is approximately that of codeine for the relief of pain. Fifty mg of propoxyphene is equivalent in analgesic effect to two to three aspirin or to 32 mg of codeine. Propoxyphene is often seen as Darvon Compound®. This is a mixture of propoxyphene and aspirin. These are efficacious drug combinations for the relief of mild pain. They do little good for the relief of severe pain. Indeed, of late, there has been speculation as to whether most of their effect is due to the aspirin in the mixture. However, it seems likely that propoxyphene, ethoheptazine, or codeine would each combine with aspirin in about the same sort of way producing a stronger analgesic. Personally, I prefer the use of codeine-aspirin combinations. They are well understood, effective, reliable, and cheap. Since these drugs have a very low potential for physical dependence, they don't worry me much.

Pentazocine

Pentazocine (Talwin) is an opiate of a rather different sort. It is an opiate, but comes from a very different type of opiate series from morphine. It is used as an analgesic for moderate pain. Although people can come to seek pentazocine regularly, it does not cause a true opiate dependence. Drug-seeking behavior is relatively rare with pentazocine. Less than one hundred cases have been reported for all the millions of doses that have been administered. However, pentazocine does generate some problems. First, it is as depressing to the breathing center as is morphine, when given in a dose that would yield an equal degree of pain relief. Thus, we still have the problem of a potential for overdose in patients for whom any lowering of breathing is hazardous. Second, pentazocine seems to have a ceiling effect at about 20 mg injected drug for analgesia. If you give a dose above this level, pentazocine causes nightmares, hallucinations, and all sorts of unpleasant feelings in people. Thus, it can be used in the relief of moderate pain, but we cannot raise the dose to a high enough level to obtain the full relief of pain that can be obtained by other opiates such as morphine, heroin, or meperidine.

Conclusion

The intent of this book is not to discuss drug abuse per se. Rather I wish to speak of the good that drugs do for mankind and to point out some of the hazards of incorrect use. Consider the great number of people throughout history who have obtained relief from suffering. It is deplorable that some people have harmed themselves by taking too much opiate, too often, and too long. But that certainly does not make me think less of the good that opiates have done for literally millions upon millions of people. For those who are interested in looking into the problems of opiate dependence in greater depth, I would suggest that you write to the Queen's Printer in Ottawa, Canada, to obtain the book *The Interim Report of the Commission for Inquiry into the Nonmedical Use of Drugs*. It is inexpensive and authoritative. Alfred E. Lindsmith's book *The Addict and the Law* and Seymour Fiddle's *Portraits from a Shooting Gallery* can also help give you a perspective on this problem.

Ergotamine and Migraine Headaches

Ergotamine (Gynergen, Ergomar) is not really an analgesic. However, it is used, usually in combination with caffeine (Cafergot, Migral), to relieve migraine headaches. It cannot be called an analgesic since it will work only with true migraine headaches and for no other kind of pain, not even other types of headaches.

A migraine headache is caused by spasms of the blood vessels of the head. Ergotamine and caffeine, if taken immediately at the beginning of the headache, constrict the blood vessels to eliminate the spasms. Ergotamine is so effective that if the headache doesn't go away, you can be fairly sure it is not a true migraine headache.

The usual dose of ergotamine and caffeine is two tablets, each containing 1.0 mg ergotamine and 100 mg caffeine, taken at the first sign of attack. One additional tablet is then taken each half hour until a maximum of six tablets has been ingested. Suppository and injectible forms of these drugs are available if nausea prevents oral administration.

Serious side effects are as low as 0.01 percent of all cases when ergotamine is used properly. However, almost 10 percent of all patients may have some nausea even at the proper dose. Weakness in the legs, numbness and tingling of the fingers, muscle pains, and a rapid heartbeat are also common, but not serious, side effects. These are caused by the constriction of the blood vessels throughout the body as well as in the head.

Fatal poisoning can result from as little as 26 mg of ergotamine taken orally over several days. This is why the drug must be treated as a potentially dangerous poison and overdose carefully avoided. Ten tablets per week is considered the maximum safe dose.

Anti-inflammatory Analgesics

There is a group of drugs that are specifically used to relieve the pain of inflammation in joints due to arthritis, gout, and similar disorders. They have only minor actions as analgesics but due to their ability to reduce inflammation in joints they can dramatically relieve pain caused by inflammation. Since their side effects are more dangerous than those of aspirin, they are all obtained only by prescription and should be used with care.

The mechanism of action of these compounds is not known. Thus, I can only discuss how they are used, not how they work.

Phenylbutazone (Butazolidin, Azolid) at a usual dose of 400 mg to 600 mg per day can effectively relieve much of the pain of inflammation. This dose appears to be the ceiling effect of the drug. A higher dose causes toxic reactions without greater pain relief. It is usually taken with meals to reduce the stomach upset often associated with its use. Its time of onset is one to two hours after taking the drug and it lasts about six to eight hours.

The adverse effects associated with phenylbutazone are both unpleasant and frequent. Side effects are noted in 10 to 45 percent of all users. In 10 to 15 percent they may be severe enough to discontinue the medication. These side effects may include edema, nausea, stomach upset, diarrhea, dizziness, inability to sleep, nervousness, blood in the urine, blurred vision, and allergy.

Two other drugs that act in a similar, but not in an identical, manner to phenylbutazone are oxyphenbutazone (Tandearil, Oxalid) and indomethacin (Indocin). Both of these also often have a number of similar unpleasant side effects.

Generally, these anti-inflammatory agents should not be taken for more than two weeks at a time.

Drugs for Gout

Gout is an inflammatory disease that is caused by the overproduction or misutilization of uric acid by the body. Crystals of uric acid settle in the joints causing an arthritic-like condition. There are three drugs specifically used to reduce the inflammation of gout by their effects on uric acid. These chemicals are useful only for the pain and inflammation of gout and no other type of pain or inflammation.

Colchicine (ColBenemid) acts by reducing the body's inflammatory response to deposits of uric acid crystals in the joints. It is the drug of choice for an acute gout attack. Colchicine is so effective that if it does not work then the inflammation of the joints is probably not gout. At its usual dose of 1.0 mg to 1.2 mg every two hours for a total dose of 4 mg to 10 mg it will stop the gout attack in twelve to seventy-two hours. It can also be used prophylactically at a dose of 0.5 mg to 2.0 mg every night to prevent gout. Unfortunately, the effective dose and a dose that will cause stomach pain, nausea, vomiting, and diarrhea are very close. Also, daily doses accumulate so that one should not take it for long in very high doses. Fatalities to this drug have occured at doses as low as 7.0 mg but people have survived larger doses.

Allopurinol (Zyloprim) acts on gout by preventing the formation of uric acid in the body. Its main use is in the prophylactic treatment of chronic gout. At its usual daily dose of 200 mg to 600 mg it is easily tolerated. About 3 percent of patients may react with a mild drug allergic response when taking allopurinol. Since attacks of gout can break through allopurinol therapy, colchicine is often used in conjunction with allopurinol.

Probenecid (Benemid) acts by increasing the excretion of uric acid via the kidneys. In the process of filtering out various chemicals from the urine the kidneys reabsorb necessary body chemicals. Probenecid inhibits the reabsorption of uric acid. For the treatment of gout the dose usually given is 0.25 gm daily for the first week, following which 0.5 gm is administered twice daily. In some patients the dose may have to go as high as 2 gm a day. Probenecid is usually well tolerated, but about 2 percent of persons taking it will have some gastrointestinal upset. Drug allergies are possible but rare. Huge overdoses can kill.

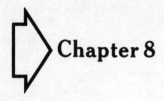

Chapter 8

Hormones

Hormones are chemicals that the glands in the body produce and that are secreted directly into the bloodstream. The term "hormone" comes from the Greek word *horme,* meaning energy. These various chemical secretions were originally conceived as giving the body energy and causing its activation.

There are a number of hormones that are used pharmacologically, that is, manufactured outside the body and taken in, rather than being made within the body. However, only four types of hormones will be discussed here since the others are relatively rarely given. The ones we will discuss are insulin; the hormones that are related to the inflammatory response, specifically adrenocorticotropic hormone (ACTH) and cortisone; thyroid hormones and the female sex hormones, estrogen and progesterone.

▶▶▶ FEMALE SEX HORMONES

Menstruation

To understand the use of the female sex hormones estrogen and progesterone you must understand the normal function of these chemicals in the body. These two hormones are produced in the female ovaries. They begin to be produced in quantity in the female just before puberty. Their production causes the growth of the female sexual characteristics and aids in the development of that delightful, but intangible, quality of the female we call femininity. The female menstrual cycle is controlled by estrogen and progesterone. During the first part of the cycle, the ovaries begin to secrete estrogen in small quantities and, with time, ever-increasing amounts. Secretion continues until three days before the onset of menstrual bleeding. Estrogen secretion causes a filling out of the breasts and the preparation of the uterus for the implantation of an egg, if fertilization occurs.

About three days before the egg is released by the ovary (ovulation), progesterone starts to be secreted by the ovary. This secretion causes an elevation in temperature that is detectable. This phenomenon gives rise to the use of temperature measurement to establish the time of egg release in the female. This is the basis of the rhythm method of birth control.

Three days before menstrual bleeding occurs, secretion of both estrogen and progesterone is abruptly terminated. Following the cessation of secretion of these hormones, the uterus undergoes changes that include the sloughing of some of the outside layer of the uterus and the rupture of small blood vessels that are coiled in the uterus. It is the rupture of these blood vessels that produces the blood flow in menstruation. All of the changes that take place in the uterus during the whole menstrual cycle are a result of the presence or absence of the two hormones, estrogen and progesterone. This has been proven in many studies using baboons after their ovaries had been removed. These animals were able to have normal menstrual cycles induced when the hormones were given in the correct dose and at the correct phasing. First, the estrogen level must build up, then there must be the additional secretion of progesterone along with the estrogen, and finally an abrupt cessation of both. Three days later menstrual bleeding will occur.

Interestingly, humans and a few baboons are the only mammals that have a menstrual cycle. Many animals have what is referred to as ovulation bleeding, which is a small amount of blood flow at the time of ovulation, but they do not have a true menstrual cycle. At this time, no one knows of what use the menstrual cycle is to the well-being of the body. Still, some physicians are a little bit afraid of interfering with the menstrual cycle by chemical means for fear that it might be useful to the body in some way that we don't yet know.

Menopause

Although possible at nearly any age, but generally in the forties, the "change of life," called climacteric or menopause, occurs for the female. When this occurs, first progesterone ceases to be secreted. Then, the estrogen production also starts a slow decline that can last for many years. The symptoms of menopause, such as hot flashes, irritability, sweating at inappropriate times, have been shown to be directly related to the lower amounts of estrogen secretion in the female. Thus, they can be corrected by an administration of estrogen from an outside source.

Estrogenic Chemicals

A number of chemicals have the same type of activity as estrogen though they do not have the same chemical formula. For example, in Australia it was found that some sheep became sterile when they were allowed to graze on pastures filled with a plant called subterranean clover. It was later discovered that this particular clover had a chemical in it that acted in the body like estrogen. The sheep had found a natural contraceptive.

Of these estrogen-like chemicals, one is of particular importance. It is diethylstilbestrol. This chemical is particularly important since it is a highly effective estrogenic agent. It is effective by mouth and, in a single dose, works longer than other estrogenic drugs since it is metabolized more slowly by the body. This means that a cheap, plentiful supply of an orally active estrogenic substance has been found. Previously, when natural estrogens from animal sources had to be relied upon, they were very expensive and shortlived in their activity. Now a number of cheap, effective diethylstilbestrol derivatives are commercially available.

The main estrogens that are presently commercially available are diethylstilbestrol, estradiol, ethinyl estradiol or mestranol (Demulen, Estinyl, Loestrin, Norlestrin, Ovral, and others), conjugated estrogens (Evex, Premarin), chlorotrianisene (Tace), quinestrol, and estradiol valerate. Each of these varies in potency. The most commonly used estrogen is also the most potent. Ethinyl estradiol, or mestranol, is effective at doses from 0.01 mg to 0.5 mg.

Various compounds that have progesteronic effects exist. However, the most common of the progesterones are progesterone (Duphaston, Proluton), ethisterone, medroxyprogesterone (Provera), hydroxyprogesterone (Delalutin), norethindrone (Norinyl, Norlestrin, Ortho-Novum), chlormadinone acetate, ethinylestrenol, norethynodrel, ethynodiol diacetate, and dimethisterone. Each of these varies as to the necessary dose, that is, its potency. The most common, norethynodrel, is usually given in doses between 2.5 mg and 10 mg.

Often an estrogen and a progesterone are given together in a tablet. This is the usual mixture found in contraceptive pills. Different varieties of these pills vary in the particular estrogen or progesterone used or in the dose of each, but their actions are all generally alike. Some common combinations are: norethynodrel as the progesterone plus mestranol as the estrogen (Enovid); norethindrone plus mestranol (Ortho-Novum, Norinyl), ethynodiol diacetate plus mestranol (Ovulen, Metrulen), ethinylestrenol plus mestranol (Lyndiol), norethindrone acetate plus ethinyl estradiol (Norlestrin), medroxyprogesterone plus ethinyl estradiol (Provest), megestrol acetate as the progesterone plus ethinyl estradiol (Volidan), and norgestrel plus ethinyl estradiol (Ovral). Finally, there are a few combinations in which estrogen is taken alone for fourteen to sixteen days and then a combination of estrogen plus progesterone is taken for five or six more days (C-Quens, Narquen, Ortho-Novum Sq, Oracon). This administration pattern more closely resembles normal bodily hormone production. However, no evidence seems to indicate any particular advantage to this sequencing of the hormones. Indeed, some evidence suggests problems associated with this approach. Also, data suggest this approach may not yield quite the 100 percent protection from pregnancy as does the continued dose of combinations of estrogen and progesterone at an adequate dose. These "sequential" type drugs have been removed from the market.

Therapeutic Uses of Female Hormones

A number of therapeutic uses exist for either the estrogens alone or the estrogens in combination with progesterones. One provides relief from the symptoms of menopause. Women of menopausal age, like everyone else, can have lots of symptoms that have nothing to do with hormones. However, for those symptoms of hormonal change, for example, "hot flashes," treatment with estrogen is specific and effective. The dose generally has to be determined by trial for each individual. For example, with diethylstilbestrol, between 0.5 mg and 2 mg daily may be taken orally for effective relief. The usual course of therapy is to take estrogen every day for four weeks, then stop taking it for one week. Menopausal symptoms will usually not recur in this week off the drug. This approach is usually used as therapy for a few months. Then, the estrogen is slowly tapered off.

This pattern of drug administration helps the woman overcome the discomfort, anxiety, and difficulties of the initial period of menopausal symptoms. On the other hand, estrogen therapy can be maintained for life. There is a series of problems that are associated with the continual declining levels of estrogen after menopause, such as increased likelihood of heart trouble (women become as susceptible to heart attack as men), a regression of the female sex characteristics, that is, the breasts become smaller and pubic hair sparse, and there can even be a softening of the bones. These problems can be eliminated with estrogen. However, because of recent evidence, many physicians are resistant to the idea of the continuous use of estrogen therapy for life after menopause. This reluctance is related to new data on adverse effects that have been associated with long-term therapy with estrogen. I will discuss these later.

Another condition that is strikingly improved by estrogens is painful menstruation. It has been found that estrogens given every other menstrual cycle will relieve most of the severe cramping that is sometimes associated with menstruation in some women. It is necessary to continually repeat the estrogen therapy every other menstrual period.

A third therapy with estrogens is the suppression of acne. Unfortunately, this can only be used with females since a male will develop some of the female sexual characteristics if given an amount of estrogen adequate to suppress acne. Most males don't like that. Also, estrogens have been proposed for the prevention of heart attacks since pre-menopausal women have so many fewer heart problems than men of the same age, but again, the dose of estrogen necessary is so great that it causes a feminizing effect upon a man so that the approach is useful only in post-menopausal females.

Oral Contraceptives

The greatest single use of estrogens and progesterones is as oral contraceptives. The initial studies by Rock, Pincus, and Garcia conducted in Puerto Rico found that by giving an estrogenic plus a progesteronic substance for twenty to twenty-one days then stopping, three days later menstrual flow would start. After the cessation of menstrual flow this hormone administration cycle was begun again. These investigators found that when the drug was used consistently, there was essentially 100 percent effectiveness in the prevention of pregnancy. Precisely how this contraception comes about is subject to some question. Probably, at the dosage used for most women, the effect of these pills is to inhibit the release of the natural hormones from the pituitary gland in the brain that are necessary to allow ovulation to occur. However, if the dose of hormones is too low to prevent ovulation, it could still prevent pregnancy by interfering with implantation of a fertilized egg into the tissue on the wall of the uterus. Thus, although the probability is that these drugs act, in most cases, in most women, by the prevention of the release of an egg from the ovary, it is also possible that, in some cases, the hormones cause abortion of a fertilized egg by making the tissue of the wall of the uterus incompatible with the implantation of the fertilized egg. The difficulty of determining precisely how these drugs work has contributed to some of the ethical problems that have surrounded the use of oral contraceptive drugs. People have differing beliefs regarding the morality of preventing ovulation versus aborting a fertilized egg. In any specific instance, you can't be sure which event occurred to prevent pregnancy.

Adverse Effects of Female Hormone Use

Taking these substances produces immediate undesirable effects in some women. These undesirable effects are quite frequent but generally quite mild. Further, they tend to go away within the first few months of using these pills. The unwanted effects are occasional vomiting, headache, discomfort in the breasts, and a gain of weight associated with the retention of excess water. Many other side effects have been reported, but in controlled studies it has been found that these were due more to expectations or worries of the women reporting them than to the actual effects of the drug.

There has been a question, due to the use of these chemicals on a mass basis, of the possibility of serious complications following their prolonged use. The first of such concerns was cancer. Estrogens, in a few animal species, when injected under the skin, in very high doses, can produce a form of cancer. However, at this time, there is no evidence that any form of malignant disease has a higher incidence of occurrence in women who use oral contraceptive drugs than in those who do not. In the case of post-menopausal women a different story is emerging. New data suggest that use of estrogen can increase the risk of cancer in the uterus and the breast. These studies suggest an increase from 1 in 1,000 to about 5 in 1,000 in cancer where estrogen is taken for long periods of time.

Second, more recently, there have been reports that contraceptive pills may add to the risk of disease due to blood clots, either in the peripheral veins or in the head. Studies even seem to suggest that women with blood type A, as opposed to other blood types, may have a greater incidence of these clots. This evidence has been very difficult to evaluate for accuracy. All the evidence is from the past. We haven't yet tried to predict the future likelihood of incidence of this disease. Past data suggest there might be 1.3 deaths per hundred thousand pill users versus 0.2 deaths per hundred thousand for non-pill-users per year. On the other hand, there has been no increase in the overall number of deaths from this type of disease since 1965, when the contraceptives were begun to be used on a widespread basis. The possibility does exist that contraceptive pill use could cause a slight rise in deaths due to the formation of clots in females. On the other hand, we have to weigh against this the fact that there is a risk of death due to pregnancy. Death due to pregnancy, from all causes, is 22.8 per hundred thousand per year. Thus, it is many times more dangerous to become pregnant than it is to take the pill in regard to possible death. I suppose all we can say is that we are not sure whether there is a slight increase in the possibility of deaths due to the formation of blood clots in users of the oral contraceptives. But we can say, with a great deal of assuredness, that the chances of death from pregnancy are a great deal higher for women who do not take the pill and who become pregnant. There is no other evidence to suggest any other serious implications for the long-term use of estrogen and progesterone as a contraceptive. I suppose everyone runs a little bit scared when dealing with chemicals that have become as widely used for contraception, over as long a period, as estrogens and progesterones. These discussions deal only with the question of contraception from a health standpoint, not the various ethical problems that can be raised about the use of these compounds.

▶▶▶ INSULIN AND DIABETES

It is estimated that there are about three million diabetics in the United States today. Of these, four out of five are over forty-five years of age and 85 percent are either overweight or have been severely overweight in their recent history. Unfortunately, only about half of these diabetics have been detected and are under the care of a physician. This lack of detection is due to the fact that many people have only mild diabetes. It may produce no symptoms or be of a level of severity that causes only fatigue, loss of weight, excess drinking of water, and overeating but is not severe enough to cause a diabetic coma. Diabetes is also related to many other medical disorders, particularly heart trouble. So it is dangerous. Great effort is now being made to detect unfound diabetics by the simple, effective method called the glucose tolerance test.

Diabetes is caused by an underproduction by the body of the hormone insulin. Insulin is produced by specialized cells in the pancreas. Normally, these cells respond to the amount of sugar in the blood that circulates through the pancreas. When the sugar level starts to go up, greater amounts of insulin are secreted into the bloodstream. The effect of insulin is to enable the body to use sugar in the blood as a source of energy and to slow the use of stored fat as a source of fuel. Thus, the secretion of the correct amount of insulin by the cells in the pancreas is essential for the maintenance of the correct balance in the use of fats, proteins, and sugars as fuels by the body. When a person is diabetic, the cells in his pancreas do not produce an adequate amount of insulin to adjust the correct balance of sugar, fat, and protein utilization. This causes a condition in the body in which higher and higher levels of sugar are present in the blood, since it isn't being used as a fuel, even to a level that sugar starts to overflow from blood into urine. At the same time, the burning of fat in the body is accelerated. This produces an excess of acidic components in the blood. A highly acidic blood will develop. It is this high level of blood acidity that can cause diabetic coma.

People going into a diabetic coma are usually confused or drowsy or unconscious, with dry skin due to a loss of water from the body, with heavy labored breathing, and a sweetish smelling breath (it smells like acetone). If they are untreated they face the possibility of death. Since diabetes can start at any time of life, people who have abdominal pain, nausea, weakness, find themselves drinking excessive fluids, have a lot of skin infections or similar symptoms certainly should check with a physician to get a glucose tolerance test to determine whether they have a maturity-onset diabetes.

Insulin Therapy

The purpose of therapy with insulin is to replace the hormone that is lacking in the body due to the inadequate production of insulin by the cells in the pancreas. Since the discovery of insulin by Best and Banting in 1922, it has been the best studied and most useful hormone to be given as a pharmacologic agent. Its use has undoubtedly saved the lives of millions of people.

In the treatment of diabetes with insulin a number of factors must be considered. First, the control of sugar intake by a carefully regulated diet is probably essential for the well-being of a diabetic. In many cases of mild diabetes, dietary control alone is adequate to keep the blood sugar at an appropriate level and to yield an acceptable rate of utilization of sugar in the body.* Second, since insulin must be given at least daily for a prolonged period of time, the patient's exact dose must be regulated as his body undergoes changes in his own rate of insulin secretion, diet, work load, and emotional status. Emotion causes the release of large amounts of sugar into the blood from the liver.

Generally, the physician will start therapy with a short acting form of insulin injection, good for three to six hours. However, after the patient has become stabilized onto a dose schedule that takes diet, work, and excitement into account, he will probably be given a longer acting form of insulin. New forms of insulin have been developed, such as protamine insulin zinc, that can last as long as thirty-six hours. These types of insulin have the obvious advantage of reducing the frequency of injections that a person must give to himself or have given to him. Unfortunately, insulin is only absorbable when it is given by injection. Pills don't work.

The major problem associated with insulin use is its potential for overdose. When insulin is given at too high a dose, or if a second dose is given too soon after a previous injection, or if not enough sugar is eaten to balance the insulin, too much insulin will be in the bloodstream. This causes a condition of too low a blood sugar level as insulin causes the blood sugar to be used as a fuel. Very low blood sugar, called hypoglycemia, results in a rapid heartbeat, high blood pressure, sweating, dilated pupils, mental confusion, loss of memory, and if low enough, coma. On the basis of observation alone, it is very difficult to know whether a person has too high a blood sugar and is in a diabetic coma, or has too low a blood sugar and is in an insulin coma. Certainly, this is not a decision any

* Although most authorities agree that detailed attention to diet and careful control of blood sugar are essential in diabetes and will help prevent serious complications, this has never been proven to be true. A few doctors feel that as long as a diabetic feels well, it doesn't matter how much sugar he spills out in his urine. However, most people will feel safer being careful.

amateur should attempt to make. It is difficult enough for a physician under the best of circumstances. Generally, he will check by determining the amount of sugar in the blood by chemical test to be sure. If a person has a low blood sugar, due to too much insulin, another dose of insulin might kill him. On the other hand, if a person is in a diabetic coma, due to a high level of blood sugar, the administration of insulin would lower blood sugar and save him.

Another problem associated with both types of coma, insulin and diabetic, is that they involve mental confusion and loss of memory. Thus, a patient who has forgotten to take his insulin shot or a patient who has accidentally received an overdose of insulin often will not be able to remember what happened. For this reason, about 50 percent of the cases of overdose of insulin or of diabetic coma are not reported in time, resulting in the death of the patient. This is why it is wise for insulin-using diabetics to wear a Med Alert tag and to have their friends and relatives aware of their condition. Then, if they do go into a coma, someone will seek immediate help from a professional.

Oral Drugs for Hypoglycemia

Recently, a series of orally effective drugs have been developed for the control of diabetes. Examples of these drugs are tolbutamide (Orinase), acetohexamide (Dymelor), tolazamide (Tolinase), chlorpropamide (Diabinese), and phenformin (Meltrol). These drugs were greeted with great rejoicing by patients who saw a chance to throw away their hypodermic needles. Unfortunately, some of the original reasons for rejoicing have turned out not to be as true as we could have hoped. Many cases of diabetes are not controllable by the oral drugs. These patients still require insulin. These are people whose pancreatic cells can no longer be stimulated to produce insulin. All insulin must come from an external source. The oral antidiabetic agents act by stimulating the cells in the pancreas to produce more insulin. If the pancreatic cells just won't produce insulin at all, these drugs can't work. The oral antidiabetic drugs have been of aid, however, in certain types of diabetes in which the cells of the pancreas are still capable of production but are sluggish and unresponsive to the trigger of circulating blood sugar. These drugs, coupled with strict dietary control, are particularly useful when using a needle to inject insulin is such a stress for the patient that it causes great discomfort. Also, there are patients whose diabetes could possibly be controlled by diet alone but who won't stick to their diets. The oral drugs help these patients burn off some of the excess sugar they eat.

Recently, one study suggested the possibility that the use of oral antidiabetic drugs increases the incidence of heart trouble. This study has been subject to much controversy in the medical profession. It is impossible at this time to tell whether to believe the results of the study or not because of flaws in the way it was done. However, it does add one more factor that the physician must worry about when he's trying to balance the delicate mechanisms involved in the body's burning of just the right amount of sugar, fat, and protein in a person whose body can't adjust itself without help. Phenformin has just been withdrawn from general use due to instances of death due to over-acidity of the blood.

▶▶▶ ANTI-INFLAMMATORY HORMONES

The odds are that you will never have to take adrenocorticotropic hormone (ACTH) in your life. On the other hand, it is fairly likely that sometime during your life you will receive cortisone, either as an injection, as a capsule, or as an ointment. In order to understand cortisone, you have to understand what ACTH is and how it works.

ACTH is a hormone produced by the pituitary gland in your brain that directly controls the secretions of the adrenal glands that, in turn, produce cortisone. The physiological significance of the adrenals was first understood in 1855 when Addison described a disease that resulted when the adrenals were destroyed. With this disease, one loses the salt and sugar from the body. However, it was not until the 1930s that large enough quantities of the chemicals produced by the adrenal glands were available to allow cortisone, and similarly acting chemicals, to be used for the treatment of inflammatory conditions, such as allergies, arthritis, asthma, or the disease named for Dr. Addison, adrenal insufficiency.

The pituitary is a gland, about the size of a small nut, in the base of the brain. This tiny gland is the master regulator of the other glands of the body. It secretes at least fifteen known hormones that regulate the flow of hormones from other glands. ACTH is released by the pituitary at a fairly steady rate all the time. However, it does undergo a variation in its secretion during each day, with the highest concentration of ACTH being found in the blood in the morning and lowest in the evening. Further, ACTH is released when you're anticipating something exciting about to happen and under conditions of emotion, loud sounds, or pain. All of these will cause an increased amount of ACTH to be released from the pituitary. This variation in ACTH flow is so well documented that its measurement can be used to judge your level of emotion, or the level of stress to which you have been subjected. ACTH which is released from the pituitary into your bloodstream circulates to the adrenal glands, which lie just above your kidneys. Here ACTH acts to release a variety of hormones from the outside portion of the adrenal glands. For our purposes, we will consider only one particular kind of adrenal hormone, the glucocorticoids, of which cortisone is the best example.

One of the effects of the release of cortisone from the adrenal glands, when stimulated by ACTH, is the suppression of the release of any more ACTH from the pituitary. This entire system, with ACTH controlling cortisone and cortisone controlling ACTH, is a negative feedback system. It is typical of the type of control that exists throughout the body. The control principle is like a thermostat regulating a furnace if you liken the pituitary to the thermostat and the adrenal gland to the furnace. As the temperature goes down, the thermostat turns on, causing the furnace to produce heat. Then, the heat from the furnace circulates back to the thermostat to turn it off when an appropriate heat level is reached. Similarly, various emotions and sounds, or stressors, trigger the pituitary to release more ACTH. This, in turn, through its action on the adrenals, causes the release of cortisone, which is like the heat. The cortisone circulates back up to the pituitary to cause the pituitary to turn off its secretion of ACTH. By using this principle of negative feedback, the body keeps itself adjusted to just the right level of cortisone necessary for the maintenance of good health. Many other bodily functions, for example, temperature, blood acidity, insulin secretion, and so on, also use a negative feedback system to maintain just the right level of activity. The body is well organized to take care of itself under most conditions. This is why we speak of "the wisdom of the body."

Cortisone-like Chemicals

Hormones of the cortisone type have a number of other biological functions besides the regulation of their own output rate by their effects on the pituitary's secretion of ACTH. They influence the way your body burns protein, fat, and sugar, help to regulate your temperature, and control inflammatory reactions. The natural chemicals of this type are cortisol or hydrocortisone (Cortef, Cortifoam, Cortril, Hycortol, Hydrocortone, and many others) and cortisone (Cortone, Neosone). Synthetic chemicals that act like these hormones are prednisolone or prednisone (Delta-Cortef, Betapar, Hydeltra, Meticortelone, Meti-Derm, Paracortol, Sterane, Sterolone, Hydeltrasol, Deltasone, Deltra, Meticorten, Paracort, Medrol), triamcinolone (Aristocort, Kenacort), paramethasone (Haldrone), betamethasone (Celestone), and dexamethasone (Decadron, Gammacorten, Hexadrol).

The effects of all these substances are virtually identical, so I will discuss cortisone only, to simplify matters. First, cortisone mobilizes protein in the body to be used as a fuel. Fat metabolism is also increased to provide extra energy. Cortisone activates your emergency energy mechanisms. This increase in the utilization of the energy sources of your body by cortisone allows for a high level of muscular activity when you need it suddenly. Second, high cortisone levels in your body, either from an outside source or from your own adrenal glands, aids your blood circulatory system in maintaining an adequate blood flow to working muscles. It also helps your heart pump a larger quantity of blood. Third, cortisone causes an excitation of your brain so it also is working in high gear. This is manifested as a good mood, restlessness, alertness, and insomnia. Fourth, cortisone causes a reduction in the heat, swelling, redness, and pain in tissue associated with injury, infection, or allergy. It is this last effect that is usually the basis for therapy with cortisone.

Cortisone Therapy

The primary use of cortisone, or other members of this family of hormones, is the temporary reduction of the pain and discomfort associated with an inflammation. Regardless of whether the inflammation is in the joints, as in arthritis, in the throat, as in bronchial asthma, on the skin, as with sunburn, eczema, psoriasis, or allergies, or in the eye due to some virus infections, cortisone will reduce the inflammation. It doesn't cure anything, but it does make living with the disorder easier. Cortisone can be given by injection, sprayed on as an aerosol, rubbed in as an ointment, or swallowed as a capsule. It is effective and absorbed by all routes.

During the course of therapy with cortisone one should start with a very low initial dose. Then, only gradually, increase the dose as slowly as possible. The reason for this approach is that administration of cortisone from an external source causes your pituitary to cease its production of ACTH. This, in turn, stops your body from producing its own cortisone. In other words, administered cortisone acts just as the normal hormone of the body would in regulating ACTH secretion by negative feedback. This interference with the production and secretion of ACTH over a prolonged period produces a situation in which the pituitary becomes almost incapable of producing its own ACTH. Then, the adrenal glands also become unable to produce natural hormones. Disuse causes the adrenals to become ineffective. You become truly physically dependent on external cortisone since your body has stopped producing it and can't produce it effectively anymore. If you suddenly try to stop taking cortisone you won't have any in your body and your body will have no ability to produce it. Physical dependence on externally administered cortisone has developed. This can be life threatening. When using cortisone for a short period only, it is a very safe drug. Even very high doses hardly ever cause any problems at all. It is only during prolonged use, that is, more than a few weeks, that difficulties can arise due to the suppression of ACTH.

In rheumatoid arthritis you can become very severely ill with fever, swelling of the joints, and intense pain. Relief is worth the problems of chronic cortisone therapy. Once you embark on cortisone therapy, however, it may have to be continued for life. For this reason, the initial dose is kept very small because the dose needed for partial relief will increase with time, that is, tolerance develops. In arthritis, cortisone acts directly to suppress the inflammatory process in the joints. It reduces the swelling and stops the deposits of the materials that surround an inflamed area. It stops the increased blood flow and the migration of white blood cells to the area. It does not inhibit the release of histamine but does block many of the actions of histamine. These actions point out another possible problem with the use of cortisone. The hormone is stopping the body's protective response to infection, that is, inflammation. Inflammation is useful if you have invading germs. When cortisone is given, the body is less able to protect itself against a real infection. Therefore, in the disorders of inflammation without germs, such as arthritis or an allergy, cortisone produces relief by blocking the inflammatory process. On the other hand, if you have an infection somewhere in your body, cortisone will block the protective actions of inflammation at the site of infection.

In a bronchial asthma attack the administration of cortisone can be lifesaving. It is very helpful in terminating an acute attack and relieving the disability of chronic bronchial asthma. To stop an acute attack, cortisone is usually given at 50 mg to 100 mg by intravenous injection over an eight-hour period. Sometimes cortisone is given in a spray inhaler. For the long-term reduction of the problems of bronchial asthma, generally the drug prednisolone is given by mouth at 5 mg to 10 mg per day in divided doses.

Skin disorders are sometimes treated with creams, aerosols, or lotions that contain cortisone. In severe cases of various kinds of rashes involving itchings and scalings of the skin, for example, poison ivy or psoriasis, a typical prescription might be a 1 percent hydrocortisone ointment applied two to five times daily. The effectiveness of this therapy is sometimes enhanced by wrapping a piece of plastic around the area so that the cortisone is better absorbed. Unfortunately, it is not only better absorbed into just the local skin area, where it will dramatically reduce inflammation and pain of these skin disorders, but is also absorbed into the bloodstream. Therefore, we have the same problems as with oral or injected cortisone. If it is used for a long period of time both tolerance and dependence can develop. Prednisolone by the oral route is also used for severe rashes.

The prolonged use of cortisone in a lotion is possibly one of the more dangerous therapies. People don't seem to realize that if something is spread on the skin it can be as dangerous as when taken orally or by injection. If they receive a tube of cortisone ointment for a skin rash, they may continue to use this ointment even though the skin rash has gone away and their physician has told them to cease using it. This is a mistake for two reasons. First, when a physician prescribes cortisone ointment for the skin, he first has decided that it is a noninfectious condition. Therefore, the cortisone will not be harmful to the body's defense mechanisms against an infection that should be suppressed. Second, he does not plan on long-term use. These creams are relatively safe for short-term use. By short-term, I mean up to a couple of weeks. On the other hand, if the person decides to continue to use the ointment he may be making a mistake. Rashes due to infection look a lot like rashes that are not due to infection. If a person suppresses his body's defense against infection, he could cause the spread of the disease through his body, making the condition much worse. Further, if a cortisone cream is used over long periods of time one has the danger, due to the absorption through the skin, of causing a malfunction of normal glandular activities. A further complication of cortisone use is that it does cause people to have a good mood as well as suppressing inflammation. Thus, people become not only physically but also psychologically dependent upon the drug. They seek it to maintain their good mood. Though incidents of complete physical dependence on cortisone are relatively rare, when it does occur the complications in the body that can result make it at least as dangerous as opiate dependence. The odds of death upon abrupt withdrawal of cortisone in a dependent person are relatively high unless careful medical supervision is available. Once again, we see that cortisone, when used properly, can reduce the pain of arthritis and bursitis, can save lives in bronchial asthma, reduce the problems of chronic bronchial asthma, and is great when used for noninfectious inflammations of the skin. Yet, it can be dangerous when used for inappropriate conditions, such as infections, or used in too great a dose, too often, for too long.

▶▶▶ THE THYROID AND THYROID-AFFECTING DRUGS

The secretion of the thyroid gland is a hormone called thyroxine. This hormone regulates the rate at which your body burns energy. Its release is controlled by pituitary hormones and also by the amount of thyroxine already in your bloodstream. Thus, a negative feedback system exists for thyroxine just as in the case of ACTH and cortisone.

An important part of the thyroxine molecule is iodine. Most of your body's need for iodine is for the production of thyroxine. If you don't live close to the sea, where your iodine requirements are met by products from the sea, or if you don't use iodized salt, your body can become short of iodine. If this occurs you can get a large swelling of the thyroid gland called a goiter. In the absence of adequate iodine the thyroid swells due to excessive activity trying to make thyroxine without iodine. However, since there is little true thyroxine produced, the negative feedback circuit doesn't stop the gland. Thus it keeps right on trying to produce more and more hormone. As little as 100 mcg of iodine, added per 1 gm of salt or some other supplement, will prevent the development of a goiter.

Hypothyroidism

When the thyroid gland does not develop in babies, a condition called cretinism develops. The baby is dwarfed, inactive, uncomplaining and listless. Its face is puffy and the tongue and lips are enlarged. The skin is yellowish and dry. This is coupled with apathy and mental retardation.

In an adult, low thyroid activity produces myxedema. In this condition the person's face is puffy and pale. The skin is cold and dry. Speech is slow and impaired. All activity of the body is slowed down.

The therapy for lowered thyroid activity is to give thyroxine. This is usually accomplished by taking pills composed of dried thyroid material from animals. These materials go under the names of thyroid powder, thyroid pills, sodium levothyroxine, or sodium liothyronine. The usual dose of a thyroid preparation is 120 mg to 180 mg per day. However, this dose has to be adjusted to each person's needs. Thyroid products are used to cause the shrinking of the thyroid in goiter. Milder forms of hypothyroidism can also be treated with these preparations. The only problem that has been associated with taking thyroid preparations at the proper dose is possible heart trouble from an overstimulation of the heart.

Hyperthyroidism

If a person's thyroid is overactive he becomes hot, flushed, overactive. His heart rate is fast. He has anxiety, insomnia, muscle weakness, increased appetite, and sometimes a protrusion of the eyes. This is called Graves' disease or Basedow's disease. The treatment for this condition is either surgery to remove part of the thyroid or one of the drugs that interferes with the production of thyroxine. These drugs prevent the incorporation of iodine into the molecules of thyroxine. The usual drugs used for this purpose are propylthiouracil, methylthiouracil and carbimazole. The usual dose of propylthiouracil is 100 mg every eight hours. However, sometimes higher doses are needed.

The adverse effects of the thiouracil drugs are rash, pain and stiffness in joints and, occasionally, drug allergy. These effects occur in between 3 and 7 percent of people using the drugs. The adverse effects are usually mild.

Since the drugs have no real effect on the disorder within the thyroid itself, they must be taken for long periods of time. If treatment is stopped the problems recur. Luckily, often the thyroid gland will cure itself during therapy. Then the drugs can be stopped without a recurrence of symptoms.

A different approach to treatment is to use radioactive iodine to kill some of the cells in the thyroid, but this treatment is too specialized to be considered in this book.

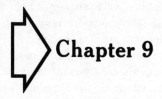

Chapter 9

Tranquilizers, Muscle Relaxants, and Anticonvulsants

Every year in the United States over ninety million new prescriptions are issued for tranquilizing drugs. This may seem like a tremendous number of prescriptions, and some people have used this number as evidence that we are becoming a drug-ridden society. On the other hand, it has been established that over seventeen million people in the United States suffer from some degree of mental illness. For example, a survey showed that on the island of Manhattan, 25 percent of the people surveyed suffered from an emotional problem severe enough to incapacitate them from full, effective functioning. Further, an analysis of the prescription data shows that most of the people who take tranquilizing drugs don't do so on a chronic basis. Rather, they take the drugs for short periods of time, a few weeks to a month, during particularly turbulent times in their lives. This indicates that, on the whole, the prescription and use of tranquilizer drugs is meeting a real need of the people of our country as we live in the harassed, polluted, noisy, plastic, tension-laden civilization we have created. Ours is an artificial life-style created by civilization. Our bodies and brains were never geared to live this way by the developments of evolution. It is not surprising then that our brain chemistry occasionally needs support from outside chemicals to get us over some of the rough spots in our lives.

Tranquilizers are generally placed into one of two major classes. Major tranquilizers, which are often used in the treatment of severe mental disorders, and minor tranquilizers, which are used predominantly by people who are not severely troubled but who do need a mild relaxant, an anti-anxiety drug, to help them through a particularly bad time in their lives. These classifications are not completely accurate. Some of the drugs generally used in the more severe forms of mental disorder also have utility in milder problems. Also, in some cases, the minor tranquilizing substances can be useful in the treatment of hospitalized patients who have more severe disorders.

For both types of tranquilizers the major effect achieved is to calm the person without producing sleep. The ideal tranquilizer would be one that reduced mental anxiety without interfering with mental functioning or producing sleep. Unfortunately, no such drug exists. All tranquilizers induce some degree of interference with mental functioning and, at higher doses, tend to produce sleep. The distinction between a tranquilizer and a sleeping pill is that the tranquilizer produces a calming effect at a dose low enough so that sleep or drowsiness is usually not produced. Thus, in discussing these drugs, we must be very careful to consider the dose of the drug. These drugs can be calming with little drowsiness if used at the right dose, but as the dose is increased, all of these drugs produce interference with thinking, loss of coordination (staggering), alcohol-like intoxication and, finally, at a high enough dose, sleep.

▶▶▶ MAJOR TRANQUILIZERS

Most major tranquilizers fall into two general groups, phenothiazines and butyrophenones. There are a number of individual drugs of each group but, for simplicity, I will discuss only one of each type: for the phenothiazines, chlorpromazine (Thorazine), and for the butyrophenones, haloperidol (Haldol). Both of these drugs have the common property of acting as antipsychotics, that is, in persons with severe mental disorders, particularly schizophrenia, they will reduce the difficulty experienced in thinking and will be calming. Both drugs reduce the occurrence of hallucinations and often eliminate them. It appears that the brain of a person with schizophrenia is always going at top speed. Because of this high level of brain activity these people have lost their ability to concentrate selectively and filter out relevant from irrelevant information. This is sort of like a motor going at full revolutions per minute all the time and the gears can't be changed. Both the phenothiazine and the butyrophenone drugs allow the slowing down of an overactive brain to cause a better focus and control of attention. The calming effect produces a more efficient brain.

Phenothiazines

The first phenothiazine to be discovered was chlorpromazine. It was discovered in France during the search for new antihistamine drugs. Chlorpromazine is a slight chemical variation of the antihistaminic drugs. Chlorpromazine itself is somewhat antihistaminic. The investigators noticed that this drug, in a low dose, caused people to become less emotional and less bothered by emotion-laden situations. They reasoned that if they gave this drug to people who were overwrought, who had disturbed and bizarre behavior, it might modify their reactions. They tried the drug on hospitalized mental patients. The results were dramatic. A chemical means had been found to treat the mentally disturbed. Patients who had been acting bizarrely and hallucinating, who were completely incommunicative, suddenly became calmer. They could communicate to some degree. Their behavior became less bizarre and they ceased to hallucinate. Initially, this led people to think that a true cure for mental disorders had been found. More recently, most specialists have come to believe that while the drug certainly improves the condition of a mentally ill person, it usually does not produce a total cure. However, drug therapy does produce a far better level of functioning by the patient than could have been hoped for before the discovery of these drugs.

If chlorpromazine is given to a normal person who is not agitated or disturbed in a dose of 50 mg to 100 mg, the person will become a bit sleepy and emotionally less responsive to his environment. This blunting of emotions is the specific effect of this drug, differing from a hypnotic effect by not producing sleep at this dose. In mentally ill people tremendously high doses of this drug are sometimes needed to produce the same sort of calming effect, perhaps 1000 mg a day. This is an excellent illustration of how a drug interacts with a person's situation at the time the drug is given. If the person is already calm and a calming drug is given, a very low dose will take effect. On the other hand, for a person with schizophrenia who is running at mental top speed, even though it is not apparent, it may take a tremendous dose of drug to produce even a small degree of calming.

When a person continues to take chlorpromazine on a daily basis, the sedative effects that cause sleepiness become tolerated, but the calming effects on the hallucinatory, bizarre, or disordered behavior continue. This is a case in which tolerance is beneficial. It eliminates one of the less desirable properties of the drug and leaves the desired calming effect intact. Further, even if a person is sedated by chlorpromazine, his state differs from the intoxicated form of sedation produced by sleeping pills of the barbiturate type or with alcohol. There is little staggering or dizziness and very little incoordination. The person can be aroused by important environmental events. In this regard, the sedation much more resembles the drowsy state caused by the antihistamines from which chlorpromazine was derived.

The probable way chlorpromazine works is by blocking the flow of information from the sensory nerves of the eyes, ears, and nose from going into the sleep center, part of the brain that controls the activation level of the brain. There appear to be separate nerve fibers that branch off from the nerve input of the main sensory organs. These nerves go to the sleep center of the brain. It is at this point that chlorpromazine acts. The drug does not directly depress the cells of the sleep center, as do the hypnotic drugs, but blocks the passage of input stimuli to it from the main sensory nerves. Thus, stimulation from the environment can still get through to the brain but will have a less arousing quality. A second means by which chlorpromazine may work is by blocking the sympathetic nervous system, possibly reducing the action of norepinephrine in the brain. It is sort of opposite in action to the cocaine-like stimulants. These two mechanisms of chlorpromazine, taken together, seem to explain the blunting of emotional reactions, while, at the same time, not producing sleep as do the hypnotic drugs. A recent theory has been proposed to account for the actions of all the major tranquilizer drugs. According to this theory there is a chemical in the brain called dopamine that stimulates some of the centers of the brain that control emotion, that stimulates nausea and vomiting, and that inhibits some special types of muscular activity. The major tranquilizers block dopamine's action. This theory could account for the effect of these drugs on mental illness and on nausea, and could also explain why high doses of the drugs given for a long time can lead to certain involuntary movements. More definitive data are needed, but it is certainly an attractive theory.

Another action of chlorpromazine that has proved to be quite important is its effect upon the mechanism in the brain that controls nausea and vomiting. Chlorpromazine is one of the most effective drugs we have for the prevention of vomiting. It and other phenothiazines were mentioned in the chapter on stomach drugs. It or related drugs are often used in the vomiting of pregnancy, or in gastrointestinal disorders in which vomiting can actually be life threatening due to excessive water loss.

Chlorpromazine is remarkably free of the common adverse effects. This is a great advantage since people who have mental disorders often have to take the drug for life. The lethal dose is very high, probably in the realm of 10,000 mg, whereas the effective dose for the normal person is 50 mg to 100 mg and for the mentally ill the dose might be up to 1,000 mg per day. Further, these seems to be little evidence that phenothiazine drugs induce any physical dependence, as do the hypnotic drugs such as barbiturates and alcohol. They do not cause any intoxication or heightening of mood. Indeed, a normal person has a rather "blah" feeling after taking them.

There can be some problems associated with the phenothiazines. Sometimes a toxic reaction can occur. They can cause damage to the liver. This liver damage may result in jaundice, which is the result of an impairment in liver function. Jaundice causes a yellowish color to the eye and to the skin. Luckily, this effect is rarely serious or persistent. Also, at very high doses, a number of the chlorpromazine-type drugs will cause tremor and convulsions. Lowering the dose or adding an anticonvulsant drug can resolve this problem.

Chlorpromazine-like drugs can cause neurological side effects. These include muscle stiffness, acute spasms of neck and mouth muscles, and a "restless leg" condition. All these respond well to antitremor drugs like benztropine mesylate (Cogentin), trihexyphenidyl (Artane), or diphenhydramine (Benadryl) and can also be avoided by lowering the dose of chlorpromazine.

Recently, it has been observed that a few patients, who have been taking drugs like chlorpromazine for a period of years, develop chronic, abnormal movements of the mouth area or of the hands and feet. These sometimes go away after the drug is stopped, but sometimes the movements persist for months or years. So far, this appears to be an unavoidable penalty attached to an otherwise very useful group of drugs. Other problems that can sometimes result from chlorpromazine-like drugs are skin reactions. An allergy response with itch, flare, and wheal occurs in about 5 percent of people who take the drugs.

The dose required for any given person will depend upon which effect is to be achieved. To stop vomiting, generally an injection of 50 mg is adequate but much higher doses can be used, if needed.

The injection route is used in vomiting because of the problem of not knowing how much has been absorbed, if any. However, chlorpromazine is easily absorbed by the stomach so it is usually given in pill form to patients suffering from a mental disorder, generally at a beginning dosage of 50 mg three times a day by mouth. If that doesn't work, the dose is increased until the desired effects are obtained.

Some of the phenothiazines that you might commonly find used are promazine (Sparine), triflupromazine (Vesprin), fluphenazine (Permitil), fluphenazine enanthate (Prolixin Enanthate), perphenazine (Trilafon), prochlorperazine maleate (Compazine Maleate), prochlorperazine edisylate (Compazine Edisylate), trifluoperazine (Stelazine), thioridazine (Mellaril), and acetophenazine (Tindal). These drugs vary in potency: fluphenazine is effective in as low a dose as 0.25 mg, chlorpromazine is the least potent. Promethazine (Phenergan) is a phenothiazine used with analgesics as a sedative, as an antihistamine, and to stop nausea.

One thing that should be emphasized, these drugs are useful in a number of conditions besides severe mental illness. I mentioned, for example, use in nausea. There are also other situations in which these drugs are used, for example, with children who are agitated or with elderly people who find their environment too disturbing for their taste, and in other conditions in which the person is not mentally disturbed but does need to have some relief from the impact of an environment.

Butyrophenones

The butyrophenones, as characterized by haloperidol (Haldol), are relatively new. They have been in use for just a few years in the United States. They differ from the phenothiazines chemically but in the majority of actions seem to be similar to the phenothiazines. For example, they block the effects of environmental activation of the brain, and they block the secretion of stress hormones by the body. For the most part, they are also similar in terms of their toxicity and side effects. The usual dose of haloperidol is between 0.5 and 20 mg orally, so they tend to be like the more potent of the phenothiazines. Another form of butyrophenone that is becoming popular is droperidol (Inapsine, Innovar). This drug is used, along with an opiate analgesic, as a special form of relaxation–pain reducing combination for operations.

There are other drugs that differ from phenothiazines and butyrophenones in specific characteristics but, for the most part, act somewhat the same. These are not common enough for us to discuss in detail. However, in case you run into them, a couple are chlorprothixene (Taractan) and thiothixene (Navane). Reserpine (Serpasil), a drug usually used to treat high blood pressure, has some weak chlorpromazine-like actions.

▶▶▶ MINOR TRANQUILIZERS

The minor tranquilizers are more similar to the hypnotic drugs than are the major tranquilizers. These drugs are used to overcome the excessive anxiety that is sometimes generated in our lives. They help calm us so we can be better able to handle emotion-laden life situations. They help us sleep at night and reduce undesirable levels of worry and tension that occur in the daytime.

Carbamates

There are many minor tranquilizing drugs available, but of all of these there are only two major ones. The first carbamate developed was meprobamate (Miltown, Equanil), by Frank Berger in 1954. He was attempting to find a long-acting muscle relaxant. Berger was impressed by the fact that meprobamate could cause relaxation at a dose that would not cause sleep. Indeed, at the usual dosage taken of 400 mg four times a day, no impairment can be found in any normal functioning, that is, in mental ability or ability to perform tasks. At the same time, the drug causes a mild reduction in anxiety generated by highly emotional situations. A person may be more capable of coping with emotion-laden situations when taking this drug. However, when you take a dose of between 800 mg and 1600 mg at one time, some degree of intoxicant-like impairment begins to occur. It is very difficult to show meprobamate to be different from a barbiturate sleeping pill when you get to these higher-than-usual dose levels.

We really don't know how meprobamate works on the central nervous system. It inhibits a variety of functions in the brain, but, as yet, we have not pinned down which specific actions are associated with its tranquilizing effects. The actions on the person are very dependent on the dose taken. When you're taking the drug in the usual therapeutic dose range of 400 mg four times a day, there is very little change in the brain action. But as you get to between 800 mg and 1600 mg at one time, the actions of meprobamate resemble those of the hypnotic drugs, which cause depression of the brain. To characterize this drug you could say that meprobamate is like a hypnotic, except that at a low enough dose it has a calming effect that can be separated from intoxication and sleep. The dose held at just the right level brings tranquilization with little sedation.

Meprobamate is also a muscle relaxant, particularly if the muscle tension is associated with nervousness and anxiety.

Meprobamate has a fairly high therapeutic safety ratio. Successful suicides with the drug are quite rare. It takes a great deal of the drug to cause death. This is a marked advantage over the barbiturates. However, meprobamate can cause death by a slowing of breathing if a high enough dose is taken. Also, allergic reactions occur in about 0.2 to 4 percent of people who take the drug. The most general complaint of people taking the drug is a bit of sleepiness and drowsiness. Sometimes, to help overcome this sleepiness, a small dose of amphetamine or caffeine is given along with the meprobamate. It helps to overcome the tiredness but there is still a calming effect if the doses of the drugs are just right.

Meprobamate combined with either alcohol or barbiturates adds up in effect. This makes it potentially dangerous if you try to take tranquilizers and sleeping pills together, or to drink alcohol when taking meprobamate. These combinations can be a particular danger if you are going to be driving, since the intoxicant effect of the sleeping pills or alcohol is enhanced. Also, it is possible to develop a physical dependence when high doses of meprobamate are taken constantly for long periods of time. If a person is given a dose as high as 5.8 gm daily for even a few days, a mild withdrawal syndrome can be observed when the person is abruptly taken off the drug. However, this is many times meprobamate's normal therapeutic dose. Dependence is rarely, if ever, seen at its usual dose of 1.6 gm per day even when given every day for four to five months. So it is possible to develop a dependency on meprobamate if it is used too often and in too great a dose for too long a time. For these reasons, the dose of meprobamate is recommended not to exceed 2.4 gm daily (six of the usual size pills).

A problem with meprobamate, and with other anti-anxiety drugs, arises when used in patients who really need a different psychiatric drug. Meprobamate won't help someone who is anxious because he is developing acute schizophrenia or someone who is very depressed, agitated, and feeling guilty. For this reason a skilled doctor should decide when a person should have a minor tranquilizer, as opposed to when he should have an antidepressant drug or a major tranquilizer.

In spite of possible difficulties, on the whole, it is my opinion that the prescribing of minor tranquilizer drugs by the majority of physicians and their use by the majority of people who take them every so often is fairly good. They are used in about the right dose and at the right time to get people over some of the bad times we all have now and then. It doesn't seem to me to be beneficial or noble to suffer unnecessary anxiety that can be incapacitating. The anxiety can hinder functioning so much you can't cope with your troubles.

We might pretend individually that we can always get along perfectly well, under all circumstances, without using drugs to help our nervous systems. But humanly speaking, there are probably very few of us who can be that competent.

Sometimes, for some people, it's better to live through the suffering without taking drugs. But nobody, including doctors, is really sure when you should or when you shouldn't. It may help though, to talk it out with your doctor and see what you jointly decide.

Other carbamates that you might see are tybamate (Tybatran), carisoprodol (Rela, Soma), mebutamate (Capla), hydroxyphenamate (Listica), and ethinamate (Valmid). Drugs resembling meprobamate in effect but differing in some of their actions are buclizine (Bucladin-S) and hydroxyzine (Atarax). These drugs yield the same results that meprobamate does but differ in potency and thus are taken in differing dosages.

Benzodiazepines

The second type of minor tranquilizer that is much in vogue these days is chlordiazepoxide (Librium) or its derivatives, which include diazepam (Valium), clorazepate dipotassium (Tranxene), and oxazepam (Serax). These are called benzodiazepine tranquilizers. These drugs differ chemically and in some other important ways from meprobamate but do have the same property of producing calming effects without producing sleep at appropriate doses. They seem to be a bit more effective than meprobamate in many cases. These drugs are essentially alike. There have been few clinical studies that have shown them to be different from each other. So I will discuss chlordiazepoxide as the specimen drug of this group. The dose for these drugs is between 2 mg and 25 mg, usually given three to four times a day.

One difference between chlorpromazine and chlordiazepoxide is that chlordiazepoxide definitely blocks the arousal of the brain from direct stimulation by the sleep center. It is somewhat like barbiturates in this respect. Further, as with barbiturates and meprobamate, there is a definite sedative action from chlordiazepoxide when taken at a high enough dose. On the other hand, many of the brain changes that follow injected doses of up to 100 mg of chlordiazepoxide resemble more the changes in the brain that take place with chlorpromazine than with barbiturates. I suppose you might think of chlordiazepoxide as something between a barbiturate sleeping pill and the major tranquilizer chlorpromazine.

Chlordiazepoxide causes muscle relaxation at the usual tranquilizing doses. Also, its action is fairly long lasting. It takes up to eight hours for full onset of drug action, and its action lasts for approximately twelve to twenty-four hours. As does meprobamate, it adds up with alcohol or barbiturates to produce an intoxicated state. Therefore, it should not be taken in combination with alcohol, barbiturates, the phenothiazines, or other tranquilizing or sedative drugs. Its toxicity, in terms of lethal effects, is very low. We really can't say for sure what the true lethal dose is for chlordiazepoxide. There are no cases reported of a successful suicide with this drug when used alone. Elderly people are particularly sensitive to the intoxicating side effects of this drug. They can develop a staggering, wobbling way of walking with a constant danger of hip fracture from falling, even at relatively low dose levels. However, for most people, the therapeutic safety ratio is something over 1:3,000 or 1:4,000. It is quite a safe drug. Attempts at overdose have been tried with up to 2.25 gm. Death did not occur. This high dose level caused prolonged drowsiness and sedation but all patients were able to be roused, and were able to talk and drink. Although respiration, blood pressure, and pulse were down, they were certainly not down to the extent that would be seen in a barbiturate overdose. This is certainly a plus for the drug. It is far safer than a barbiturate. Chlordiazepoxide can cause the usual allergic rashes and other side effects found with all drugs, but these are not common.

Physical dependence is possible with the benzodiazepines. The dependence somewhat resembles that caused by barbiturates or meprobamate. However, in one study, patients received 300 mg to 600 mg per day every day for several months. This is about ten times the usual therapeutic dose. Suddenly the drug was stopped. A few of these patients had fairly severe withdrawal symptoms. Most had mild withdrawal symptoms of depression, agitation, insomnia, loss of appetite, and some evidence of mental confusion. However, it took quite a bit of drug for quite a long time for this much physical dependence to be developed. Also, generally people do not actively seek this drug, perhaps because it does not produce a "high" the way barbiturates or alcohol do. Thus, drug dependence seems a small problem and very rare in occurrence, particularly since most people taper off their dosage rather than attempting to stop abruptly.

Doxepin

A new drug has been discovered that reduces the problems associated with a differential diagnosis between anxiety and depression. Doxepin (Sinequan) is used at a dosage of 75 mg to 300 mg per day for either anxious or depressed patients. It acts almost immediately to reduce anxiety, but its antidepressant effects require two or three weeks to develop. Its adverse side effects are dry mouth, blurred vision, and constipation. Occasionally, sweating, weakness, chills, rapid heartbeat, fatigue, ringing in the ears, and rash have occurred to patients taking doxepin. It also adds its effect to alcohol, making the person who drinks along with taking doxepin very drowsy. This can be dangerous if you have to drive a car. The drug has a moderate therapeutic safety ratio; death by acute overdose will be relatively rare. We are glad to have this new tranquilizer available for treating a symptom such as anxiety, since any one type of tranquilizer will not always work for everyone. Recent studies suggest that other tricyclic antidepressants may share doxepin's effect in states of mixed anxiety and depression.

▶▶▶ MUSCLE RELAXANTS

The activity of muscle relaxing drugs is believed to relate to their ability to block certain kinds of reflexes while leaving other reflexes intact. The simplest reflex that we have is called a single neuron reflex. An example of this is the knee jerk reflex. This occurs when you are tapped just below the knee cap. It is called a single neuron reflex because when you are tapped, a signal goes from the stretch-sensitive neurons in your muscle to your spinal cord. From there, the signal goes right back down to your leg to cause it to jerk. So only one nerve is involved for the signal to come up and one to go back down. It's all controlled in the spine.

The other kinds of reflexes in the muscles are more complicated. They require a large number of nerve cells for their actions. These are called "polyneuron" reflexes. A deliberate decision on your part to move a muscle involves this type of reflex. For example, when you make a decision to move, this "will to act" is translated down to the muscles by reflexes that require a large number of nerve connections. The effect of relaxant drugs seems to be to cause a fairly severe inhibition of reflexes that are polyneuronal but to leave the simpler nerve reflexes relatively unaffected, so all complex muscle action is relaxed but the simpler reflexes needed for balance, standing, sitting erect, etc., are less affected. Notice I say relatively unaffected because there is also some inhibition of the simpler nerve reflexes as well as of the polyneuronal ones. Also, these drugs are mildly tranquilizing and sedating. Therefore, if the tension in the muscles is related to mental anxiety, the drugs also exercise some of their effects by reducing anxiety. Common relaxant drugs and their usual adult, oral doses are as follows: methocarbamol (Robaxin), 1 gm to 2 gm four times a day; styramate (Sinaxar), 200 mg four times a day; chlorzoxazone (Paraflex), 250 mg to 750 mg three or four times a day; and carisoprodol (Rela, Soma), 250 mg to 350 mg four times a day.

On the whole, the degree of effectiveness of relaxant drugs is not great compared to tranquilizers or hypnotics. You get muscle relaxation if you take meprobamate or benzodiazepine tranquilizers. Indeed, the benzodiazepines are fast becoming the drugs of choice for muscle relaxation. You also get muscle relaxation if you take barbiturates or alcohol. So, there is little advantage in using a "muscle relaxant" since, unfortunately, for all these drugs, the dose that is necessary for skeletal muscle relaxation is very close to the dose that produces sedation. Quite often it may be the sedation and tranquilization that actually give any beneficial effects that may be received. A further problem with these drugs is that quite often they are prescribed in a dose that is too low to actually give a useful effect. A great deal of the effect may be more attributable to expectations of benefit than to chemical properties of the drug at the recommended dose.

The muscle relaxants are found in both injectable and oral forms. They are absorbed fairly well from the gastrointestinal tract within forty-five minutes. Their duration of action is relatively short. They work for only a couple of hours whereas the benzodiazepine tranquilizers have the advantage of being longer lasting. The standard muscle relaxant drugs have a relatively low toxicity but can cause death by depression of respiration if given in a very large dose. This is very rare. So far, no reports of dependence have occurred for these drugs. The side effects of an undesirable type are occasional weakness, nausea, vomiting, dizziness and double vision. Also, the usual allergies can occur with muscle relaxants, though they are rare. It appears that these drugs are relatively innocuous, but they are also relatively ineffective in achieving the desired condition of muscular relaxation without the production of tranquilization or sleep. It's too bad we haven't discovered better drugs for muscle relaxation, considering the number of people suffering from low back pain, stiff necks, muscle soreness, and so on. It still seems that the best therapy for conditions of localized muscle pain is soaking with a hot cloth and some aspirin. If the muscle pain is caused by tension of an emotional origin, then the tranquilizer drugs are adequate to help produce relaxation, and they are longer lasting in their effects. Hopefully, we'll be able to come up with better compounds soon.

▶▶ ANTICONVULSANT DRUGS

Anticonvulsant drugs are used for control of epilepsy. This is a disorder that afflicts four million people in the United States through no fault of their own. It is a disease like any other disease. Luckily, now, it is usually very controllable and, indeed, curable in some cases.

Epilepsy is a general term that is used for a number of different types of disorders. However, all of these disorders have something in common. They are brief episodes called "seizures." In a seizure there is loss or disturbance of awareness, and sometimes, but not always, it is characterized by involuntary body movements called "convulsions." These terms are perhaps a little confusing. By seizure all we mean is a brief period of a loss or disturbance of consciousness. By "convulsions" all we mean is some degree of involuntary body motion. This involuntary motion can be as little as a flick of a finger or as great as the full involvement of almost all the muscles of the body.

Types of Epilepsy

The major types of epilepsy are: (1) "Grand mal," in which there is major movement of all or most of the body. This includes a loss of consciousness with jerking and loss of control of most muscles including those that control and hold in fecal material and urine. (2) "Petit mal," which is characterized by a brief loss of consciousness, perhaps just for a few seconds. Sometimes there is just a little jerk in the body, sometimes no body movement at all. (3) "Psycho-motor" epilepsy, which is characterized by confused behavior and a wide variety of other mental effects. This kind of epilepsy produces only a disturbance of consciousness. It does not produce uncon-sciousness. (4) "Diencephalic" epilepsy, which is associated with various kinds of changes in the functioning of the internal organs, for example, stomach aches. (5) "Focal cortical" epilepsy, in which the motor disturbance is confined to a small muscle group, say one arm only, or a facial tic. (6) Finally, there are various other epileptic-like symptoms that are more common; most people experi-ence them once in a while. These are minor little isolated jerks, such as those that occur sometimes when you're about to go to sleep. These jerks are of an involuntary nature. We know very little about their cause.

The Cause of Seizures

In all cases, epilepsy is associated with a faulty firing of nerves in the brain. Generally, this faulty firing of nerves starts out at one spot in the brain. It then spreads to the rest of the brain. This faulty spot in the brain is the result of either a disorder that has been present from birth or of a head injury or illness. There can be all sorts of reasons why one small part of the brain can become hyper-sensitive. This hypersensitive area will occasionally start to fire very fast, at a much higher rate than required for normal functioning. Many things can trigger this hypersensitive brain area. It could be a change in blood chemistry or blood sugars, or because of tension or fatigue. Any one of these or other causes will initiate too high a firing rate in the hypersensitive area. Next, the excessive activity in the small hypersensitive area can begin to spread to other areas of the brain, like a chain reaction with the trigger at the one hyper-sensitive area.

Everybody's brain has this tendency to spread any activity that happens in one part to other parts. However, there are also inhibiting factors in normal brain cells that prevent activity from spreading too fast. In the person who is suffering from epilepsy, it seems that the area of incorrect functioning, the hypersensitive area, is so large and fires so fast that the normal inhibitory mechanisms of the rest of the brain cells cannot stop the spread of this activity. So the high rate of firing is spread to the rest of the brain. This causes the body to jerk uncontrollably and for the person to become disturbed in consciousness or to lose consciousness altogether. If all parts of the brain are firing in a disorganized fashion, literally, the brain goes into a chain reaction similar to one in an atomic bomb. Luckily, the cells of the brain can't sustain this activity. So, as the brain cells fatigue, there is a cessation of the chain reaction and the seizure is over. Different forms of epilepsy show somewhat different patterns of brain activity but fundamentally all of them can be thought of as caused by one small, slightly damaged, hypersensitive part of the brain that fires so fast that the rest of the brain can't turn it off. This effect spreads through part or all of the rest of the brain. Then, as the brain cells tire, the seizure is over.

The ideal anticonvulsant drug would be one that is very safe in terms of its therapeutic safety ratio, that would cause no toxicity, would not cause sleep or sedation, could be taken for very long periods of time, and would control all types of epilepsy. No such drug exists at this time. However, 70 percent of epileptics can be rendered free of seizures and socially functional with current drug treatment methods. Quite often, if medication can be started when the patient is young, there is a complete elimination of seizures and the epilepsy is cured. Then no further medication is needed. Particularly at adolescence, there seems to be the possibility of an elimination of all seizure activity. On the other hand, often seizure activity will stop during adolescence even without medication, so it is hard to say that the drugs do or do not cause the cure. Thus, we can say that not only is epilepsy controllable, but, indeed, it is sometimes curable. For that matter, sometimes time alone is all that is necessary for its cure.

Barbiturates for Epilepsy

The oldest drug to be used in the treatment of epilepsy is the barbiturate phenobarbital, which has been discussed in the chapter on hypnotics. It should be noted that not all barbiturates have the property of being effective anticonvulsant agents. Phenobarbital, additionally, has the advantage over other barbiturates of being a very long acting compound. Thus, you don't have to take the drug so often. If it is taken only occasionally and the dose is controlled, excessive tolerance will not develop. The drug then can be taken for years without the development of physical dependence or excessive tolerance. Phenobarbital is usually given at a dose of 200 mg a day or less. This dose can vary quite a bit from person to person. Other barbiturates used in epilepsy are metharbital (Gemonil), mephobarbital (Mebaral), and primidone (Mysoline).

Diphenylhydantoin

Perhaps the most dramatic event in the history of the treatment of convulsive disorders occurred with the discovery by Merritt and Putnam of diphenylhydantoin (Dilantin). Diphenylhydantoin is not a sedative. Patients are able to function without any sedation or impairment of consciousness. The discovery of diphenylhydantoin sparked a new search for other drugs that might be even better for the treatment of epilepsy.

Diphenylhydantoin is particularly effective for people suffering from grand mal epilepsy. It is also sometimes useful in other types of epilepsy but does not seem to be of much use in petit mal epilepsy. Diphenylhydantoin acts by stabilizing the actions of cells in the brain and not allowing them to fire too fast. Thus, it acts to contain the overactivity of the hypersensitive area alone. This prevents the spread of the seizure to surrounding brain areas. On the other hand, it does not impair the ability of nerve fibers to carry normal impulses. It only stops them from firing too fast. It is a stabilizing drug without being an inhibiting drug for normal activity. It stops the trigger area of hypersensitive tissue in the brain from being able to detonate the rest of the brain in a chain reaction.

Usually diphenylhydantoin is given to adults at 100 mg three times a day, orally, as a beginning dose. It takes at least a few days for this dose to work its way into the body effectively. Then the physician must see whether this is an adequate dose to suppress all seizures. Generally, adults can go up to 500 mg a day without any evidence of toxicity. However, beyond this point toxicity does start to become a problem. Children under six usually require about a third of this dose. After six they can be given adult doses.

Acute overdose of diphenylhydantoin causes dizziness, nausea, and problems in vision. Chronic overdose can cause hypersensitivity that gives rise to a variety of problems from troubles in the stomach, to allergic reactions in skin, or even damage to liver and bone marrow. However, it's easy to diagnose hydantoin overdose by blood tests. The therapeutic safety ratio is quite high. Many grams of the drug have been taken in attempts at suicide but deaths are very rare. It's difficult to commit suicide with diphenylhydantoin. The problems of side effects can be fairly serious, 2 to 5 percent of the patients get rashes. In chronic use, swelling and overgrowth of the gums occur in almost 20 percent of patients. The drug is not as harmless as we would like. On the other hand, since it will abolish all seizures in 65 percent of the patients and reduces the frequency and severity of seizures in another 20 percent, it is still a godsend to an epileptic.

Other hydantoins, such as mephenytoin (Mesantoin) or phenylethylhydantoin (Nirvanol), are essentially similar in their effects. Ethotoin (Peganone) and albutoin (Co-ord) are other similar drugs that occasionally will be seen.

Other Anticonvulsant Drugs

Phenacemide (Phenurone) is a triple-action drug in that it is therapeutically effective not only against grand mal, as are the hydantoins, but also against petit mal and psychomotor seizures, for which the hydantoins don't work. Unfortunately, its toxicity to the central nervous system, liver, and bone marrow is much higher than for hydantoins. The incidence of side effects is about 17 percent in terms of psychological changes, 8 percent for stomach problems, 5 percent rash, 4 percent drowsiness, 2 percent problems in the blood, and 2 percent hepatitis. Thus, this drug is rarely used in epilepsy unless the condition has proven unresponsive to treatment with anything else. However, it is nice to have in the wings in case nothing else works.

Trimethadione (Tridione) and paramethadione (Paradione) offer more variation in the treatment of epilepsy. These drugs are selectively effective in petit mal epilepsy. Trimethadione and paramethadione both act in a manner different from diphenylhydantoin. Where diphenylhydantoin acts to contain the area of brain activity to one spot, preventing the explosive detonation throughout the rest of the brain, trimethadione and paramethadione prevent neurons within the hypersensitive area from being overactivated. They selectively block high-speed chains of impulses. They are particularly effective in controlling overactivity in the lower areas of the brain that drive the parts of the brain that govern consciousness. This is the major action of these drugs. Without an overactivity of these lower brain sites, you don't get the disturbance or loss of consciousness that characterize petit mal epilepsy.

These drugs are readily absorbed by the oral route. The usual adult daily dose is between 300 mg and 2.1 gm. The adverse side effects that commonly occur are blurring of vision when in bright light and drowsiness. This drowsiness can sometimes be overcome by taking amphetamine or another stimulant drug at the same time. This addition of a stimulant does not interfere with the effectiveness in the control of epilepsy. Rarely, but sometimes seriously, problems can occur with skin rashes, blood changes, or damage to kidneys and liver.

There are some relatively new anticonvulsant drugs. They were developed with the desire to find other effective drugs for petit mal that had less toxicity than the ones previously discussed. These are phensuximide (Milontin), methsuximide (Celontin), and ethosuximide (Zarontin). While they do seem to achieve good results in the control of petit mal, it is questionable whether they are any less toxic than trimethadione or paramethadione. Some physicians feel they are safer.

In some ways the field of anticonvulsant therapy is one of the truly great successes in modern pharmacological research. On the other hand, the ideal anticonvulsant drug has not yet been discovered. Quite often it is necessary to carefully work out the individual dose and the individual drug best for a given patient. Quite often more than one anticonvulsant must be used to get just the right effect. Yet, when we consider the horror and shame that was the lot of an epileptic or of his family just a few years ago — his constant fear of having a seizure and all the things that this fear prevented him from doing in life — we must be grateful that most cases can be controlled or cured. The next time someone starts complaining about our "drug culture," think about the epileptic and how much he has benefited from the development of new drugs.

Chapter 10

Antibiotics

Antibiotics are the most often prescribed drugs in medicine. A few years ago these were referred to as the "wonder" drugs. It is interesting to consider the changes in the public's views that have led us from the era of the "wonder drugs" to the era of "wonder about drugs." Truly, these drugs are one of the most remarkable scientific advances that man has ever made. The use of antibiotics, plus large-scale immunization and sanitation, has extended man's life and wiped out most of the diseases that have plagued man throughout the centuries. Unfortunately, other countries in the world do not have the advantages of nearly universal immunization, careful sanitation, or an adequate supply of antibiotics that we enjoy. Thus, many of the diseases that we consider rare are still rampant in other parts of the world.

Antibiotics interfere with the reproduction, multiplication, and life of germs. In order to understand the way these drugs work and some of the problems that can be generated by their use it is necessary to consider the nature of germs. First, let us think of germs in the aggregate, a germ colony, or, if you will, a germ "city." Germs are individual organisms that must eat, drink, reproduce, compete with each other, and defend themselves against enemies in the same sense that you and I must. However, they live at a remarkably high rate of speed. If you think of individual germs in a colony as a group of individual people in a city, you might liken the growth of a germ colony in twenty-four hours to what has happened to the city of Chicago in the last one hundred years. Also, in the same way that refuse from the city of Chicago pollutes and poisons the Great Lakes and surrounding areas, refuse products from a colony of growing germs are poisons that can pollute and destroy your body. A local infection is the result of this poisoning and pollution in a localized area. If the germs spread throughout your body, the local infection becomes a general disease.

A germ's lot is not an easy one. In trying to grow in the thriving activity of its colony, it must compete with each of its neighbors for the food, water, and other resources it needs in order to continue to grow and reproduce itself. Also, there are many natural enemies of germs in your body. There are other, benign germs that do not cause illness that are normal residents of your body. These benign germs compete with the disease germs for the same resources of food and water that your body is providing. Further, there are specialized cells and mechanisms within your body that are constantly trying to attack, wall off, and destroy the disease germ colony. It is only when the disease germ colony overwhelms the natural defenses of your body that you develop an infection. Usually, your body fights back effectively.

In the fight against infection, a germ may also be thought of as an individual, not just as a whole colony of germs in growth. Even individual germs of the same type differ from one another. The way in which individual germs of the same type differ that most concerns us here is their ability to resist the action of an antibiotic. Each germ has its own individual sensitivity to the effects of an antibiotic — its own individual dose-response curve. For some individual germs the curve is well to the left, indicating a high degree of sensitivity. For some it is well to the right of the average, indicating a high degree of resistance to the specific drug. This susceptibility or resistance of the individual germ cell to a specific antibiotic is a genetic characteristic that is transmitted to the germ's offspring.

All these considerations enter into the determination of the dose and administration schedule of antibiotic necessary to kill a particular germ colony. When you're sick you take a dose of an antibiotic. This dose is distributed throughout your entire body. It is metabolized and detoxified by your body. Part of it is stored in various organs. Finally, some small amount gets to the germs. The amount of drug that gets to an individual germ is dependent on the amount of drug that you take, your body's metabolism of the drug, and the number of germs among which the drug is divided. Thus, when you take a drug, you take a given dose. That dose is many, many times subdivided before it gets to an individual germ cell. The amount of drug available to poison an individual germ might be called the dose per germ. Whether the dose per germ of the drug harms the germ cell or not depends upon the type of drug and the resistance of the germ cell to that drug at that dose.

▶▶▶ THE ACTIONS OF ANTIBIOTICS

An antibiotic can have one of three kinds of action on a germ cell. (1) It may be below the threshold dose. In this case it does absolutely nothing to the germ cell. (2) At a higher dose, it can stop the reproduction of the germ cell, that is, it acts as a contraceptive for the germ. (3) At a still higher dose, the drug kills the germ. The ideal of antibiotic therapy is to establish a dose per germ in your body at a level high enough to either stop the reproduction of the germs so that your body mechanisms can kill them or to directly kill the germs. Yet, the total dose should not cause you too many unpleasant side effects.

Different antibiotics have different effects upon different types of germs. Not only are there differences in the sensitivity to an antibiotic among individual germ cells within a type, but there are also vast differences in sensitivity among types of germ cells. For example, a drug effective against an infection of gonorrhea might not be effective against typhoid fever. Further, most antibiotics now available have very little effectiveness against most disorders caused by viruses. If you take an antibiotic to cure the common cold or other upper respiratory infections caused by viruses, you're wasting your time. You may even cause yourself harm.

The Misuse of Antibiotics

Now that we've laid out what a germ is and how it lives and grows, let's consider the different ways in which antibiotics are used or misused, so we can see the consequences of both correct and incorrect use. First, take the situation in which an antibiotic is taken for a type of disease germ that is highly resistant. What will happen? Probably, you will take a dose that will be too low, in the dose per germ, to get to the threshold level. This means the germs will go their merry way, growing and reproducing, without any interference from the drug. On the other hand, the benign germs, natural to your body, which are competing for the same food and water resources with the disease germs, may be killed by that drug at that dose. In this case, the disease germs will be able to grow more easily than before. Now they do not have competition from the benign germs, which the antibiotic has killed. So, by taking an antibiotic that is not poisonous to the disease germs but that is poisonous to benign germs, you're actually aiding the growth of your disease.

Too low a dose of antibiotic per germ can also be taken when you wait too long after the onset of the disease to use an antibiotic. The antibiotic is divided among all the germs that are there. If you have waited until the germ colony has grown very large, then logically, for a given total dose of drug, the amount of drug per germ will be lower since there are more germs. This total dose may be below threshold dose and again be ineffective in killing the germs causing you the problem. This is why, if an infection is well developed, it is necessary to take a much higher dose of the antibiotic than you normally would take if you had caught the disease in its early stages. If this happens your physician will often try to get a lot of antibiotic into you quickly, for example, by injection. He may also give you another form of antibiotic, such as a pill, to continue for a longer period. In this way the drug gets to the infection as rapidly as possible before it grows too large, and also the drug stays in your body long enough to kill all the germs.

If you stop taking an antibiotic too soon problems can occur. When you take an antibiotic at an adequate dose, generally you will feel better in about three days. By this time most of the disease germs will have been eliminated. It is quite common for people to stop taking an antibiotic because they feel better. However, as I mentioned before, individual germ cells differ in their resistance to the drug. Therefore, the least resistant germs are killed off first. As the number of germs declines, if you continue to take the same total dose, the amount of drug per germ increases as the number of germs decreases. This can be compared to a holdup involving twelve accomplices. Your share would be so much. If you start eliminating accomplices one by one, your relative amount of the loot goes up proportionately. The same principle applies here. As the drug is working, it first kills the least resistant germs. So the amount of drug per germ, like the amount of loot, goes up. Therefore, the most resistant germs are killed as the dose per germ increases. As you continue taking a drug at a fixed level, the actual amount of drug per germ is constantly increasing. If you cease to take the drug after only three days, what you've done is to kill off those germs that are least resistant to the drug, but there may be a number of germs left that are the most resistant. These are the ones that take a lot of drug to interfere with or kill. Also, you will have killed off a lot of the benign germs that are normal to the body. This leaves a group of germs that have genetic capacity to resist the drug, living in an environment where they don't have to compete with weaker germs of their own kind or with benign germs. They're going to have a heyday. They will proliferate and pass the quality of resistance to the drug to their offspring. You now have a reinfection with a type of germ that is highly resistant to the antibiotic. If you try to take the antibiotic again, the dose necessary to achieve a dose per germ to kill this resistant form of germ may very nearly be the dose that will kill you. Perhaps even worse is the fact that you can now infect other people with this resistant form of germ.

The development of antibiotic resistant germs has caused tremendous problems. We now have a number of drug resistant germs due to misuse of antibiotics. It is sometimes very difficult to kill these new germs without getting up to doses of antibiotic that may harm or even kill the patient. This developed because people took either: (1) an inadequate dose of antibiotic so just the weak germs were killed; (2) they didn't continue taking the drug long enough to really eliminate the whole germ colony, or (3) in some cases, they waited too long to begin antibiotic therapy so that it became almost impossible to eliminate all the germs, and only the most resistant ones lived. For these reasons, when you have inadequate therapy with an antibiotic, you're not only harming yourself, you may be harming the rest of us too by creating resistant germs. Let us hope we can continue to invent new antibiotics as fast as the drug resistant strains of germs are developed due to the misuse of antibiotics.

Let us review the common misuses of antibiotic therapy. *First*, their use in the treatment of fevers of obscure origin. Many things can cause fevers: hormones, allergies, a failure to sweat, virus infections. If the fever is not serious or life threatening, it is usually inappropriate to treat it with an antibiotic until it has been established what particular kind of germ you have, if any, and what drug the germ is sensitive to. This involves a little extra bother and a day or two more of suffering for you, but at least you know you're going to get the right drug. *Second,* the use of the wrong antibiotic for a particular germ; the drug won't affect the germ that is causing the problem but will affect other benign germs. *Third,* an inadequate dose of drug; resistant germs are developed. *Fourth,* the use of a drug for infections, such as viruses, that just aren't affected by antibiotics, for example, measles, mumps, the common cold, flu, polio. *Fifth,* stopping the drug before you're supposed to. You may feel better in three days but you should take the drug for at least seven to ten days to ensure that all the germs are killed, not merely those that have the least resistance to the drug. *Sixth,* and perhaps the worst, is the use of antibiotics when it is not known what disease is being treated. The fact that your neighbor is suffering from symptoms not unlike those you had, and for which the doctor gave you a particular antibiotic, does not mean that he has the same sort of germ. If you give him an antibiotic that has little or no effect on his particular germs, you may be making your neighbor's infection much worse. Unless you can examine the particular germs and determine exactly what kind they are and then run antibiotic sensitivity tests to find which drug will best kill them, don't prescribe for your neighbor. Too many diseases have many similar symptoms. The average person just isn't able to diagnose either for himself or his neighbor. The fact is that we are all being endangered by the development of resistant strains of germs of a number of very dangerous diseases because of the acts of a few people.

Sulfa Drugs

Antibiotics are chemical agents which stop the growth of germs or kill them. Antibiotics are derived from living plants or animals, such as other germs, molds, funguses, or primitive plants. Sulfa drugs, technically, are not antibiotics since they are derived synthetically from chemicals, not from living organisms. However, since they are used in the same way as the antibiotics and the same general principles apply to their use as with the antibiotics, it seems best to discuss them in this chapter.

Gerhard Domagk deserves the credit for the original discovery of the sulfa drugs. For this discovery he won the Nobel Prize for medicine in 1939. He found that sulfanilamide (Prontosil) was effective in the therapy of infections. Since their original discovery, over fifty-five hundred different sulfa compounds have been produced. However, all of them work by the same means and differ only in their rates of absorption into and mode of elimination from the body. All sulfa drugs act to prevent the growth of germs. At usual dose levels they do not kill the germs, only inhibit their growth. When the sulfa drug has inhibited the growth of the germ colony, natural body mechanisms that counter infection come into action to eliminate the small, nongrowing colony of germs.

The sulfa drugs act on germs because of the way that the sulfa drug molecule appears to a germ. In order to reproduce and multiply, a germ requires the presence of a common chemical of the body called para-aminobenzoic acid.* Sulfa drugs resemble para-aminobenzoic acid. The germs mistakenly take in the sulfa drug instead of needed para-aminobenzoic acid. The sulfa drug does not act like para-aminobenzoic acid. It does not allow the germ cell to reproduce and multiply.

Not all kinds of germ cells or even all germ cells of a given type require para-aminobenzoic acid in order to reproduce and multiply. Those germs that do not require this chemical in their environment cannot be affected by the sulfa drugs. Further, in every colony of germ cells there will be some germs that have only a partial need for

---

* Interestingly, para-aminobenzoic acid (PABA) or its salts are the chemicals used in some antisunburn creams. It has the property of blocking most of the ultraviolet light from your skin, thereby preventing burning but still allowing tanning to take place. It is called a "sunscreen" in this application.

para-aminobenzoic acid. These individual germ cells, then, are more resistant to the action of sulfa drugs. This ability to reproduce with only a little para-aminobenzoic acid by some germ cells gives them their capacity to be partly able to resist the actions of sulfa. From these germs, whole new resistant colonies can develop. As was mentioned earlier, if some individual germs are resistant to a particular drug and all the other germs are killed off, then these resistant germs grow at a faster rate because there are no other germs to compete for the nutritional resources in the environment. So, if one takes too low a dose of sulfa, or takes it for too short a period of time, one can develop an entire colony of resistant germs that need little or no para-aminobenzoic acid. This new colony of resistant germs can be contagious; the resistant strain of the germ can be passed on to other people. For example, between 1941 and 1945, 70 percent of all gonorrhea cases were successfully treated by sulfa drugs. However, from 1945 to 1948 only 20 to 30 percent of all cases of gonorrhea could be cured with sulfa drugs. This shows that during the period 1941 to 1945 resistant strains of the germs developed. When these were transmitted to other people, the effectiveness of sulfa drugs for many cases of gonorrhea became greatly reduced.

Since all sulfa drugs work by the same method, if a germ is resistant to one of the sulfa drugs it will also be resistant to the other sulfa drugs. This is called cross-resistance.

The Adverse Effects of Sulfa Drugs

The possible adverse effects of all sulfa drugs are fairly similar. First, they share with all other drugs the possibility of causing an allergic reaction. With the sulfa drugs the percentage of allergic reactions is a good deal higher than for most other drugs; from 2 to 10 percent of people who take these drugs will have an allergic reaction. A second adverse effect that is specific to the sulfa drugs is their tendency to form crystals in the kidneys. Sulfa drugs are soluble in fluids to only a limited degree. Therefore, when sulfa drugs are being excreted in the urine, there is a chance that if the concentration of the sulfa drug is too high, the drug will come out of solution to form small crystals of sulfa that embed in the kidneys. These crystals block fluid flow and irritate the kidneys. They can cause permanent damage to your kidneys. For this reason, it is very important that when you take a sulfa drug, you produce an adequate volume of urine. The more urine there is, the greater is the amount of solution in which the sulfa drugs can be dissolved and the less likely it is that the drug will come out of solution to form crystals in your kidneys. You should be sure to take in enough fluid to produce 1200 ml to 1500 ml of urine every day. This requirement of a high fluid intake (several quarts of liquid each day) is more important for some of the sulfa drugs than for others, but, in general, it is good advice when taking any sulfa compound. Sometimes, to reduce the odds of having crystal formation, a combination of two kinds of sulfa drugs is used. Using different forms of sulfa can provide the high levels needed in the blood to stop an infection and still minimize the chance that the sulfa will crystallize in the kidneys.

With all the sulfa drugs, almost anything can happen as an untoward side effect. If you are using a sulfa drug and get any strange symptom at all, it is wise to quickly check with your physician because it could be a reaction to the sulfa.

Types of Sulfa Drugs

There are four kinds of sulfa drugs. These types have different rates of absorption and excretion. First, there are those that are rapidly absorbed and rapidly excreted; second, those rapidly absorbed but slowly excreted; third, those absorbed very poorly from the gastrointestinal tract when administered orally and therefore effective in controlling germs in the gut; fourth, there are a few sulfa drugs that have unique properties that make them useful for special purposes.

Rapidly absorbed and rapidly excreted forms of sulfa that are most likely to be given to you are sulfadiazine (Quinette, Suladyne), sulfamerizine, sulfacetamide, and sulfamethazine (Otocin). These drugs are quite similar. They are commonly used for treating infections of the urinary tract since they are excreted unchanged in urine. Usually, they are given as an oral dose of about 1 gm every six hours. Generally, it is necessary to maintain this dose level for at least seven to ten days in order to ensure that the germs are eliminated. These same drugs can be used for a number of other kinds of infections, gonorrhea, for example, but unfortunately, many types of infections are now resistant to them.

Some new forms of rapidly acting, rapidly excreted sulfas have been more recently developed. These are sulfisoxazole (Gantrisin), sulfacytine (Renoquid), sulfamethizole (Azotrex), and sulfamethoxazole (Gantanol). They have an advantage over the older drugs in that the percentage of people who have formation of kidney crystals is less than 1 percent. This is due to the higher relative solubility in urine of these particular sulfa drugs. However, as with all other sulfa compounds, they can cause a fair percentage of cases of allergic response.

The rapidly absorbed and slowly excreted sulfa drugs are useful when a long-term administration of the drug is needed to stop germs that are not easily wiped out. For example, some types of urinary infection are very difficult to cure and require months of therapy. To make it more convenient for the patient, it's good to have a drug that is easily absorbed by the oral route but slowly excreted so that pills can be taken twice a day rather than every six hours. However, this means that the drug is not eliminated from the body as quickly. Therefore, if you have an allergic or toxic reaction to the drugs, taking a slowly excreted type is more of a problem since the drug will be in your body for a longer time after you have stopped taking the pills.

The three common sulfa drugs having rapid onset and slow excretion are sulfamethoxypyridazine (Midicel), sulfadimethoxine (Madribon), and sulfameter (Sulla). The dose of these drugs is a bit lower since they stay in the body longer, usually about 0.5 gm twice a day. They have the same adverse reactions as the other sulfas: potential formation of crystals from urine if there is not an adequate fluid intake and about a 6 percent chance of adverse side effects of one kind or another.

There are a number of very poorly absorbed sulfa drugs that have a specific use in the preparation of a patient for surgery, when it is necessary to clean out the gut and partly sterilize it, or in the treatment of diarrhea, or running stools, caused by germs. However, these particular uses are very specialized and you probably won't run into them too often. It is interesting, however, that the lack of absorption from the gastrointestinal tract into the blood can be utilized to produce good therapy. In this case you don't have to worry about the problems of formation of crystals in the kidney or the other things that happen when the drug is in your blood. Since the drug isn't absorbed, it goes from your mouth to your rectum stopping all germ growth on the way. So, in this case, the lack of absorbability of the drug gives it its particular therapeutic utility for gastrointestinal infections.

Some types of sulfa are used specifically for eye infections. Other kinds are designed specifically for prevention of the invasion of germs into burn areas. But they are rather uncommon forms of sulfa.

In the past, sulfas have been used as creams, ointments, powders, and lotions. However, this is presently discouraged. First, placing a drug on the skin is more likely to cause an allergic reaction than any other way of using a drug. The skin is particularly sensitive to allergic response from drugs. Also, studies in World War II found that in cases where sulfa powder was dusted over wounds, often the sulfa powder would cause a scab that actually prevented the drug from getting to the germs. The scabbing made more trouble than if the wound had not been powdered with sulfa. So, on the whole, except in some rather specialized cases, the powders, lotions, and ointments made with sulfa are no longer used in good therapy.

Penicillin

The story of the discovery of penicillin is one of the most dramatic in the entire history of pharmacology. One day Alexander Fleming left a dish containing a culture of germs out on his desk. Accidentally, a small mold spore drifted through the window. It settled into the dish. Later, Fleming observed that around the spot where the mold had landed there was a clear area where all the germs had been killed. It was an exciting discovery: a substance produced by this mold could kill germs. The mold turned out to be a common bread mold named penicillin.

After its initial discovery, little attention was paid to Fleming's mold. However, during World War II a group of men came together to attempt to develop Fleming's findings into a practical therapy. First, they had to develop means by which a very pure form of the mold could be produced in large quantity. Then, they had to run all of the animal tests and human clinical studies to ensure that it was an effective means of killing germs without killing patients. By the summer of 1943, five hundred clinical cases had been treated, and our first true antibiotic had joined the armamentarium of pharmacology.

Although this is an appealing story, actually mold products have had a long history of use in medicine. In ancient days of the Egyptian Empire, wounds were treated with poultices of moldy bread. In the early 1900s investigators found that molds other than penicillin produced substances having the capacity to kill the germs. However, no one can overlook the importance of the discovery and insight of Alexander Fleming or the dedication of the group of men that followed him to produce the first true "wonder" drug.

Now, as a result of an immense amount of scientific work, there are a number of kinds of penicillin. We have even come so far as to be able partially to make penicillins artificially. The production of semi-synthetic penicillins involves adding specific chemicals to mold cultures so that different kinds of penicillin can be produced. This advance has led to the development of longer-acting penicillins, the orally effective penicillins, and the new penicillins that have the ability to kill germs that have become resistant to the older types of penicillin.

Penicillin's Mode of Action

Penicillin acts by interfering with the ability of a germ cell to maintain the integrity of the wall that surrounds it. The germ requires having an intact wall around it to protect it from elements of its environment that are poisonous to it and to allow aspects of its environment needed for growth and reproduction to pass into it. Penicillin interferes with the cell's capacity to maintain that intact wall. By making the germ cell open to chemicals that are poisonous to it, penicillin at moderate doses destroys the cell's capacity to reproduce, and at high doses can kill the cell.

Unfortunately, germs vary in sensitivity to the action of penicillin. Thus, the same problem exists with penicillin as with all other anti-germ agents. If the dose taken is not adequate enough to destroy the colony, there will be some germs present that are resistant to penicillin at that dose. These will grow to produce penicillin resistant strains. Further, some types of germs are not sensitive to penicillin at all. Also, as with all other drugs, penicillin has some adverse side effects.

The dose of penicillin and some other antibiotics is often not referred to in milligrams. Rather, if you examine a bottle, you will see the term "units." A unit of penicillin is that amount of penicillin that it takes to kill a specified number of germs The amount is determined by actually taking a sample of each batch of penicillin to see how effective it is in eliminating a number of different types of germs. All batches of penicillin are compared against an international unit of penicillin that has been established. After many years, however, we have finally obtained pure enough batches of sodium penicillin G to know that one milligram of this drug equals 1,007 international units. Now we can translate the "unit" measures to a pure measure in milligrams of sodium penicillin G. However, most generally, you will still see doses stated as so many hundred thousand or so many million units of penicillin, referring to the number of germs it will kill.

Types of Penicillin

There are a number of types of penicillin but the first discovered, classic one is penicillin G. Since penicillin G is inadequately absorbed from the gut, it is almost always administered by injection. It reaches high blood levels very quickly, in fifteen to thirty minutes, but then it begins to be metabolized very rapidly; within three to four hours after administration hardly any of it is detectable in the body. This is a quick in–quick out type of penicillin. Since one of the goals of antibiotic therapy is to get the drug in as quickly as possible, before the germ colonies grow larger, and then to maintain a high level of the drug in the body for a sufficient period of time to kill off the germs, penicillin G must be injected about every two to three hours continually. These constant injections hurt and are a bother. One way around this problem is to suspend the penicillin in oil and put it deep into the muscle instead of giving it just under the skin. The drug is absorbed more slowly when it is in oil and deep in a muscle. It seeps out into the body at a slower rate. Using this technique one can maintain an adequate level of procaine penicillin G in the body for about twenty-four hours with one injection. A good technique of therapy is to combine the two approaches, a shot under the skin and also one into deep muscle. This gets the drug in fast and also maintains an adequate dose for at least twenty-four hours. Using this approach of therapy, you will often get a dose between 300,000 and a million units of penicillin every twenty-four to forty-eight hours. Sometimes your doctor may inject a dose as high as 1.2 million units deep into the muscle to maintain a fairly high level of penicillin for ten to fourteen days.

Penicillin is excreted from the body unchanged through the kidneys. Thus, it can be a useful drug in curing kidney infections. With a dose of 100,000 units of penicillin G every three hours you can very easily get up to 1,000 units per 1.0 ml of excreted urine. Penicillin G is rapidly absorbed and rapidly excreted when injected under the skin, therefore it is a good drug to quickly get a high dose of drug into the kidneys or urinary tract for the treatment of infections in those areas.

There are various forms of administration of penicillin G. The one to be used depends on the kind of absorption and excretion rate you want. It can be carried in either an oil vehicle for intramuscular injection or a water vehicle for injection under the skin. Also, rate of absorption depends on whether the penicillin G is connected to some other kind of a molecule, such as procaine or benzathine, in order to delay its entry into the blood to give you a longer-acting substance. Some of the names that you might see for penicillin G, in one or another of its forms, are Crysticillin, Depo-Penicillin, Diurnal-Penicillin, Lentopen, and Bicillin.

A number of new penicillins have been invented that seem to act by a mechanism similar to that of penicillin G. However, they must differ in some manner from the original compound since some germs that have shown a resistance to penicillin G are not necessarily resistant to these new forms of penicillin, too. Thus, though the mechanisms of action are probably similar they could not be identical or else cross-resistance would be complete. Some of the new penicillins that have been developed are effective by the oral route and some are very long acting. A few of these new types are phenethicillin (Darcil, Chemipen, Maxipen, Syncillin), methicillin (Staphcillin, Celbenin), oxacillin (Prostaphlin), cloxacillin (Orbenin, Tegopen), dicloxacillin (Dynapen, Pathocil, Veracillin), nafcillin (Unipen), ampicillin (Amcill, Omnipen, Penbritin, Polycillin, Principen), amoxicillin (Amoxil, Larotid), hetacillin (Versapen), carbenicillin (Geocillin), and phenoxymethyl penicillin (Potassium Penicillin V, Compocillin-VK, Pen-Vee K, V-Cillin K).

Often a drug named probenecid (Benemid) is given with penicillin. This drug inhibits the excretion of penicillin in the urine. Combining probenecid with penicillin will increase blood levels of the antibiotic two- to four-fold. It does not have this effect with the other antibiotics — only penicillins. It is also used in treating gout, as was discussed in the chapter on analgesics. It can cause a drug allergic response but seldom does at its usual dose of 2g a day.

Adverse Effects of Penicillin

The incidence of adverse effects varies with the particular type, dose, and route of administration of the various penicillins. Penicillin G produces the highest incidence of adverse reactions, about 5 percent. Further, all penicillins can cause the extreme allergic reaction of shock. Shock can kill very quickly. This is why it is important for a person to know if he is allergic to penicillin. If he is, this is a drug that can kill rapidly. Unfortunately, this reaction is not too rare. About two out of every hundred thousand patients may die from an injection of penicillin. About three hundred people each year die from penicillin-induced shock. These are still pretty good odds if you're really very sick and need the drug. On the other hand, if you aren't really very sick, the odds are not so good. If you are one of those people who have an allergy to penicillin, there are other kinds of antibiotics that can be used instead of penicillin. Luckily, serious allergies are less likely to occur with the new, orally effective penicillins.

Although penicillins can cause various kinds of allergic reactions, their direct toxicity is very low. No one has ever actually determined what the lethal dose of penicillin is, it is so high. So, if you are not allergic to this drug, the chances are that it is almost impossible to poison yourself with it.

Penicillin is a useful drug in a tremendous number of kinds of diseases. However, as with all other antibiotics, it is wise always to determine the specific germ causing your trouble and whether it is, or is not, sensitive to the effects of penicillin. It is also important to be sure to get penicillin in an adequate dose, quickly enough, and for a long enough time to totally wipe out the infection. A brief listing of some kinds of diseases that generally can be treated with penicillins are bacterial (not viral) pneumonia, meningitis, streptococcal infections, scarlet fever, many infections in the heart, all kinds of gangrene, local infections such as wounds, gonorrhea, syphilis, anthrax, diphtheria, rat bite fever, and a fair number of others. You'll notice that I did not mention the common cold or other diseases produced by viruses. The antibiotics do not help them.

Streptomycin

Wonderful as penicillin and the sulfa drugs are, there are still a large number of germs that have either developed resistance to these agents or could never be affected by them in the first place. Thus, in 1944 when the discovery of the next antibiotic, after penicillin, was announced, it was a day for great rejoicing, particularly since this new antibiotic appeared to be effective in killing the germ responsible for tuberculosis. This new agent was streptomycin. Indeed, it turned out to be true that many types of germs that were resistant to sulfa and penicillin could be killed by streptomycin. Examples of the kinds of diseases that began to look very curable were bubonic plague, rabbit fever, tuberculosis, brucellosis, meningitis, and tick fever (Rocky Mountain spotted fever).

Unfortunately, though this is an effective drug, it has its hangups. First, streptomycin is not able to be absorbed by the oral route. Second, it seems to be very difficult to find variations of it that are long acting. Third, it causes an allergic reaction in about 5 percent of patients. Fourth, a serious toxicity was discovered. Nearly 75 percent of patients who were given 2 gm of streptomycin for sixty to one hundred twenty days developed fevers, difficulty in vision, difficulty in coordinating body movement, staggering, and a great deal of neurological damage. Some of these patients required from twelve to eighteen months to recover. Some never did. Even at a dose as low as 1 gm daily there was approximately a 25 percent incidence of this kind of direct toxicity for the nervous system. Further, deafness occurred in from 4 to 15 percent of individuals taking the drug for more than one week. Hearing returned when the drug was discontinued. But, in some cases where the drug was taken for longer periods of time, the deafness was permanent. A final problem is that germs can develop resistance to streptomycin faster than to any of the other antibiotics. Resistance can develop in as little as forty-eight hours. After forty-eight hours the drug may be useless.

Because of its toxicity and the rapidity with which resistant germs develop in the presence of streptomycin, it's used much less than it used to be. It is generally used only when other drugs have been tried and the particular germs are found not to be sensitive to them, and when the germs are known to be specifically sensitive to streptomycin. We are still glad to have the drug for the resistant germs and for diseases that are so dangerous the risk of damage caused by the drug is worth it. It can still be a lifesaving antibiotic with the right use.

Chloramphenicol (Chloromycetin)

Another drug that is exceedingly effective in killing germs is chloramphenicol. Yet, as with streptomycin, chloramphenicol is seldom used these days. It is effective in killing a number of germs that are resistant to other drugs. However, in addition to the usual possible allergic reactions and some nausea on initial use, this drug has one great failing. The drug can be responsible for a deterioration of the blood-making marrow in the bones. This is not a dose-dependent phenomenon but just happens in some people for reasons we don't understand. Therefore, it's like an allergic phenomenon in that it doesn't matter how much is taken, it just happens to some people. This bone marrow deterioration can be reduced, to some extent, by keeping a very careful watch on the patient, not giving the drug for too long, and avoiding repeated administrations. However, one in forty thousand people taking chloramphenicol will develop this very serious interference with the function of bone marrow. If there is an interference in bone marrow function, the red blood cells that are produced are defective — they cannot carry oxygen as they are supposed to. When this problem develops it is a lethal disorder in almost 100 percent of the cases.

Why is it then that we continue to use an agent where perhaps one in forty thousand people who use the drug will be killed? The reason is simple. We use it when nothing else will work and the disease is going to kill you anyway if something isn't done. Then, the drug is very handy — well worth the risk. An example might be typhoid. Typhoid is often quite resistant to other antibiotic agents. Chloramphenicol is very effective in killing the germs responsible for typhoid. Typhoid will kill you very quickly unless something is done. Therefore, the risk has to be considered — one in forty thousand will die from the drug. On the other hand, a higher percentage will die from typhoid if nothing is done. So you must weigh the possible benefit and the possible risk. Then, you do your best and hope. But never take chloramphenicol for a minor, non-life-threatening infection.

Tetracycline

Since the discovery of penicillin, streptomycin, and chloramphenicol a systematic study has been made of funguses, bacteria, and other living organisms that might produce drugs of use to man. From this search, one of the most significant discoveries was tetracycline (Aureomycin, Terramycin, Achromycin, Declomycin, Vibramycin, Minocin and others). This class of antibiotic compounds is so effective against a wide range of different kinds of germs that they were given the name "broad spectrum" antibiotics. Also, in many ways, the tetracyclines are safer, having fewer side effects than the other antibiotics. Thus, a new degree of safety as well as effectiveness was introduced to the field of antibiotic therapy. However, do not take this to mean that they are effective against everything or that they don't have any problems associated with their use. Over the years, there has been some evidence of the development of resistance of some kinds of germs to the tetracyclines. Also, they can cause drug allergy. The tetracyclines act on germs by inhibiting their ability to synthesize the correct kinds of protein they need to live and reproduce. The drug specifically combines with the portion of the germ cell that is responsible for guiding the germ's production of various kinds of proteins. Without the kinds of proteins that are blocked by tetracycline, the germ is unable to produce foods it needs for life and growth.

The tetracyclines are well absorbed by the oral route. Doses of between 1 gm and 2 gm a day are the usual therapeutic dose. An initial oral dose of 250 mg produces a peak drug level in the blood within two hours. This level lasts for about six hours. For this reason, the daily drug doses are usually divided — a 1-gm to 2-gm daily dose into four equal parts over the day at about 500 mg each time to maintain a constant, adequate level. An interesting problem with this drug is that the presence of milk or milk products, or of any antacids, in the stomach, will hinder its absorption into the blood. This is too bad since the tetracyclines are a bit irritant. In some people they cause nausea and indigestion. However, taking them with meals slows absorption, but also eases any stomach distress. If you take the drug at the same time that you take an antacid tablet or dairy product, there is an excellent chance that none of the drug will get into your system. Antacids and dairy products effectively block the absorption of the drug. Thus, antacids or dairy products and tetracycline should not be taken at the same time.

Most tetracyclines are extracted from the blood by the liver. There they are changed and then eliminated through the gallbladder into the gastrointestinal tract. Since little tetracycline gets into the kidneys, these drugs are not as effective as sulfa drugs for the treatment of urinary tract infections. They can be used, since a bit of the drug goes out via the kidneys in urine, but they are not as effective as other antibiotics.

Allergic reactions do occur with the tetracyclines. However, they are relatively less common than with the other antibiotics. Further, direct toxic effects are minimal except for the irritation of the stomach. Tetracyclines do have some interesting side effects that are rather different from some of the other antibiotics. One of these is a sensitivity to the sun. A patient can easily get sunburned from being out in the sun even a short time when taking these antibiotics. Further, there are some problems with injury to the liver in a few people who take the drug at greater than the usual 2-gm-a-day dose. However, this is not too prevalent a disorder. Also, they cause a change in the fats in your skin. This property makes them useful in the treatment of some cases of acne. This will be discussed in the chapter on drugs for your skin. They are seldom given to children or pregnant women since they can discolor developing teeth.

Germ resistance to the tetracyclines can develop, but it tends to be a slow process, very different from the forty-eight-hour process for resistance developed with streptomycin. The single greatest problem with the tetracyclines is their use for an infection from a germ not affected by them. It kills the benign germs, eliminating the disease germs' competition. The result of this elimination of most of the germs usually found in the gastrointestinal system is the possibility that staphylococcus or other germs can grow suddenly, and explosively, if they have a resistance to the tetracyclines. It is possible, but very rare, to die from a staphylococcal infection that is resistant to the tetracyclines because of elimination of competing germs. On the whole, however, we can be very thankful that tetracyclines were developed to add to the weapons we have to fight infections.

Antituberculin Drugs

Tuberculosis is a classic example of a disease that has been almost entirely checked by the use of drugs. It was once one of the most common of the debilitating illnesses. Now, although it is fairly common, it seldom debilitates or causes death.

Tuberculosis is caused by an infection by a specific germ and therapy depends on taking antibiotics that can inhibit the growth of that germ. The tuberculosis germ is resistant to most of the antibiotics.

The major drug used with tuberculosis is isoniazid, often abbreviated as INH (Nydrazid). This drug, at the usual dose of 300 mg per day, acts on the tuberculosis germ by inhibiting its growth. How it does this is not known. Isoniazid is easily absorbed by the oral route. It can cause drug allergic responses but they are rare. In a few people convulsions can occur. However, this is usually associated with a vitamin B_6 deficiency. Isoniazid causes the body to rapidly burn B_6. For this reason, B_6 tablets are often taken with isoniazid. Occasionally, eye problems develop with drug use. It is a good idea to have periodic checkups during isoniazid therapy.

To cure tuberculosis it is necessary to take isoniazid for at least eighteen months to two years. This is a bother. Many patients often forget to take their pills. Since drug resistant tuberculosis germs develop very rapidly, this is a very bad situation. To forget to take the drug regularly can cause the therapy to lose its effectiveness owing to resistant germs.

Because of the high instance of isoniazid resistant tuberculosis germs, it is common practice to combine another antibiotic with isoniazid to be sure the growth of as many germs as possible is inhibited. Drugs often used for this purpose are cycloserine (Seromycin), para-aminosalicylic acid (PAS), viomycin (Viocin), ethambutol (Myambutol), or rifampin (Rifadin, Rifamate, Rimactane, Rimactazid).

Other Antibiotics

There are a number of other antibiotics that have recently been developed. Each has its own particular advantages and disadvantages. However, in general, the same principles of use already discussed for other antibiotics apply to these newer drugs. Examples of these are erythromycin (Ilotycin, Erythrocin Lactobionate), cephalexin (Keflex), cephalothin (Keflin), cephaloridine (Loridine), cephaloglycin (Kafocin), neomycin (Mycifradin, Myciguent), paromomycin (Humatin), kanamycin (Kantrex), polymyxin B (Aerosporin), colistin (Coly-Mycin), vancomycin (Vancocin), cephapirin (Cefadyl), bacitracin, tyrothricin, lincomycin (Lincocin), gentamicin (Garamycin), cephradine (Asspor, Velosef), and others. Each of these drugs must be considered in terms of the specific germs that it can kill, its effectiveness by different routes of administration, the presence or absence of resistant germs, chance of infection from other, competitive germs that it doesn't affect, and allergic reactions or toxic responses.

Antifungal Agents

A number of diseases of mankind are not caused by germs but by funguses. Lately, we have developed some types of antibiotics that are effective in destroying funguses. This has been a great advance since previously fungus-caused diseases had been some of the most difficult to cure. Some of the fungal disorders are most deadly. Other types are only very common and troublesome. The deadly diseases caused by the funguses are not too common in this country but are prevalent in other countries; these include such diseases as histoplasmosis and coccidioidomycosis, lethal diseases, and we may be thankful that we have some new drugs to combat them. Two types of fungal disorders of less seriousness but greater prevalence are ringworm and athlete's foot. Though not fatal, they certainly are bothersome.

Agents that are effective against the funguses also have some degree of effect against germs, but do not affect parasites, worms, or viruses at all. Some of the common antifungal agents that are produced by living organisms, and therefore are antibiotics, are nystatin (Mycostatin), amphotericin B (Fungizone), griseofulvin (Fulvicin, Fulvicin U/F, Grifulvin, Grifulvin V, Grisactin), and tolnaftate. These are the ones you are most likely to run into. The other antifungal antibiotics are used in the rare, but potentially lethal fungal disorders. Griseofulvin and tolnaftate are used in common, but less lethal, diseases.

Griseofulvin

Griseofulvin was developed in the search for different forms of penicillin. It is produced by penicillin mold. It was discovered in 1946 to have an active effect against funguses and also against some germs. It has been found to be highly effective against a variety of diseases caused by funguses but is of particular use in curing ringworm. Ringworm is not caused by a worm but by a fungus.

Griseofulvin acts by combining with the fat in the fungus. By doing this it causes a relative increase in the protein in the fungus. This throws the metabolism of the fungus out of order and, at low doses, will cause its growth to stop and, at high doses, will kill it. This is interesting from a pharmacological standpoint since the drug is one of the few that acts by combining with the fat in a cell. Most drugs that act by combination with some part of the cell do so by combining with the protein material.

Griseofulvin at a dose of about 0.5 gm is rapidly absorbed by the oral route. It reaches a peak concentration in the blood in about four hours. From there it distributes itself through all body tissues but has the property of being attracted more to skin that is diseased with a fungal infection than to normal skin. This is, of course, a very useful property of the drug. It makes new skin or hair that grows in the body area that has previously been infected with the fungus, resistant to the disease, so that as the old skin sloughs off through normal wear and tear and old hair grows out, the new skin and hair that grow in are free of the fungus. Since it requires a considerable period of time for new skin or hair to be formed and for infected skin to be sloughed off, the drug must be taken for a fairly long time. However, symptomatic relief from the disease will usually appear after only forty-eight to ninety-six hours of therapy. It may take between three weeks to twelve months before totally fungus-free cells will appear in the skin, hair, fingernails, and toenails.

The incidence of serious reactions to this drug is amazingly low. However, a few minor adverse side effects do exist. One is a head-ache that occurs in about 15 percent of people when therapy is first begun. Generally, it is mild and disappears as therapy is continued. However, sometimes it is severe and does not disappear. There are a few other possible problems including, of course, an allergic re-sponse or excessive fatigue in a few people. It can add up with alcohol to make you drunker on less alcohol, but this is a relatively rare event. This drug is almost always used in the form of an oral dose. It is essentially ineffective when placed directly on the skin. You don't rub it onto the fungus but rather let it come from the inside to go out to the fungus.

Tolnaftate (Tinactin)

This agent was synthesized in 1960. It has been found to be a very effective agent for various fungal disorders but particularly in the treatment of athlete's foot. It has little or no effect on germs. Usu-ally, tolnaftate is directly applied to the skin area affected. A com-mon use would be to sprinkle tolnaftate as a powder on the itching, shedding skin area between your toes where the fungus is present, four or five times a day. This is one of the few antibiotics that is applied topically to the skin. This application has to be continued for a month or so and will usually rid you of the infection, but there are some types of funguses that are resistant to the drug. Finally, to this time, there have been no toxic or allergic reactions reported for tolnaftate. However, as the drug continues to be used, undoubtedly, sooner or later, somebody is going to have a toxic effect or allergic reaction to it. It always seems to happen when we think we have a totally safe drug.

Undecylenic Acid

Another drug commonly used for the treatment of funguses on the skin — particularly athlete's foot — is undecylenic acid. It is not an antibiotic since it is not derived from a living organism. It was developed for the military during World War II to help control the many fungus infections picked up by troops in the jungles. It is an effective drug for many types of fungus infections.

This chemical or perhaps a derivative of it such as zinc undecyle-nate, is usually employed as an ointment or a powder placed directly on the infected area four or five times a day. It may take months of use to totally stop an infection. No adverse effects have been reported for even very prolonged use of this drug. Often it is used in conjunction with salicylanilide or acrisorcin (Akrinol), which also act to impede fungus infections.

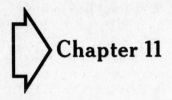

Chapter 11

Antidepressants

Last year, in the United States, over seventeen million prescriptions were issued for chemicals to alleviate the condition known as "depression." It appears that there are a great many unhappy people in the United States. This unhappiness may be so great that it incapacitates the person so he cannot function normally in his daily life. This doesn't mean that every time a person is unhappy he is truly depressed in the full psychiatric meaning of the term. It is normal for every human to have mood swings, from happiness to unhappiness, but most of us spend most of the time riding somewhere about the middle. However, during some periods of your life, perhaps due to the death of a loved one or after a loss of self-esteem, the degree and pervasiveness of sadness may become so excessive as to paralyze you from taking appropriate actions; you can become so debilitated that you cannot take the correct actions to alleviate the sadness. Further, there are some people who live for weeks, months, or years in a condition of such extreme sadness that their whole mental life is spent in a consideration of the misery of their state. It is these cases of extreme, incapacitating, enduring sadness that we refer to as "depression." It's not just that you're sad, but that you are so sad and hopeless as to impair your ability to do something about your sadness or to live a normal life. This extreme sadness leads to further misery and anguish — deeper into the black pit known as depression.

Until 1958, the only two available means for helping overcome the debilitation of depression were the use of psychotherapy and electroconvulsive shock therapy. These methods were useful in many cases in helping to relieve the depression. The use of electroconvulsive therapy is still the single most satisfactory means for relieving many of the most severe depressions. However, in 1958, Kuhn found the first of a series of drugs that could also be of benefit. He was actually studying new tranquilizers of the phenothiazine series like chlorpromazine, but he found that although one of these drugs was relatively ineffective in quieting agitated psychotic patients, unexpectedly, it did help some types of depressed patients. Further, the drug helped both the usual kinds of severely depressed people, those who were somewhat agitated, trying to fight their depression, and those who had just given up — the slowed, withdrawn, retarded depressives. This discovery led to many clinical trials of this drug, and the development of other compounds that also showed effectiveness in relieving depression, or at least improving the depression. These antidepressive drugs are called tricyclic drugs. Members of this group are imipramine (Tofranil), desmethylimipramine (Norpramin), amitriptyline (Elavil), nortriptyline (Aventyl), and protriptyline (Vivactil). Although these different drugs vary slightly in the speed with which they start to work and their potency, fundamentally, their actions are all quite similar.

From a subjective standpoint, the effect of these drugs is to take the edge off the depression. They give the depressed person a slightly greater sense of objectivity in dealing with the problems in his life. This has been referred to as "dulling of the depressive thought pattern." This doesn't mean that you can't think about your problems, but rather, that when you do think about them, they don't cause quite so extreme a sense of hopelessness. This certainly does not mean that the drugs cause happiness or elation. Far from it. They just take some of the helplessness and bitterness out of the feelings about life's problems. This then allows the depressed person to deal with the problems and gradually eliminate or forget them with greater efficiency.

In the brain the drugs act in a way that is somewhat similar to the actions of cocaine, amphetamine, and other stimulant drugs. Also, in some ways, they act something like the phenothiazine tranquilizers. First, as with the stimulant drugs, they prevent the reuptake of the chemical norepinephrine into storage sites in the brain where it is ineffective. This prevention of reuptake of norepinephrine causes a high level of free, circulating norepinephrine in the brain. The nerves activated by the free norepinephrine stimulate a number of body mechanisms. However, the tricyclic drugs differ from cocaine in that there is little evidence to suggest that they cause any extra release of the norepinephrine. Thus, the effect of these antidepressive drugs is to cause a slow, gradual increase in the amount of free norepinephrine in the brain, which translates itself, through a number of pathways, to a raised energy level and elevation of mood that can help a person cope with his problems.

These drugs also act much like the tranquilizer chlorpromazine. Similar to chlorpromazine, they cause the side effects of dryness in the mouth and lowered blood pressure. In the nondepressed person they can cause feelings of fatigue. In these ways they resemble a tranquilizer. They also help the depressed person by decreasing his anxiety and reducing his insomnia. Considering the nature of the effects caused by these drugs, they seem to be best described as a combination of a tranquilizer and a stimulant. Thus, the person with a depression gets the relaxation of a tranquilizer and, at the same time, the greater potential energy and the better mood necessary to cope with his problems.

Treatment with Antidepressants

The usual treatment with antidepressive drugs would be somewhere between 50 mg and 250 mg per day (10 mg or 50 mg tablets taken up to five times per day). Often after the first week or so of taking a tricyclic drug, the total dose can be taken at one time. This works just as well. This dose must be taken for at least a week before any drug action becomes apparent. Sometimes up to two or three weeks pass before improvement is noted. Interestingly, it often appears that people other than the patient will first notice that the drug is acting. Although life may seem the same to the person taking the drug, other people will notice that he has greater energy and vigor as well as an improved mood. He will begin to deal with the realities of his life and problems in a more adequate way. All this is noticed by others before the person, himself, feels that he is any different.

The prolonged time before the drug starts to have its effect against the depression is interesting, since the drug is rapidly absorbed by the oral route and is relatively rapidly excreted. Within four to five hours after administration, a good part of the dose of the drug is already gone. We don't know why it takes one to three weeks for the drug to start having its effect.

Each of the antidepressive compounds is different in degree of stimulation or sedation that it produces. This is a useful trait since depressed people feel differing degrees of agitation or fatigue. The most tranquilizing of these drugs is amitriptyline. Amitriptyline causes a fairly large degree of sedation and tranquilization, along with its antidepressive effects. Imipramine is about average. It produces little stimulation and also little tranquilization. The most stimulating of these drugs is desmethylimipramine. It not only causes an antidepressive effect but also stimulates the person at the same time. Thus, due to these differences, the particular antidepressive drug can be matched against the level of activity of the depressed person to help normalize his activity level at the same time that he is getting the antidepressive effects.

Adverse Effects of Antidepressants

There are some problems associated with the administration of antidepressive drugs just as with any other type of drug. First, if a person takes too large a dose, it can cause excessive excitement and even hallucinations. However, this occurs in only a small number of people and only with a relatively high dose. Second, particularly during the initial period of treatment, there are some unpleasant side effects with these drugs, such as dry mouth, constipation, dizziness, rapid heartbeat, blurred vision, and sometimes, a difficulty in urinating. Luckily, these side effects usually drop out as a person develops tolerance to them. They cease to cause any trouble after a few days or weeks of administration. However, a persistent, fine tremor of the hands and limbs can be observed in about 10 percent of people who continue taking these drugs for long periods of time. This is particularly likely in elderly patients when the dosage has reached at least 250 mg a day. Further, the drugs can produce allergic drug reactions in some people. Also, in rare cases, they can cause damage to the liver. This liver damage is first seen as a yellowing in the whites of the eyes called jaundice. This jaundice shows that the liver is not working correctly to put bile fluid out into the intestine.

A final problem with the antidepressant drugs, and one that causes many people to object to them, is weight gain. People who are taking antidepressive drugs start to eat more than they should.

This is so universal a phenomenon that unless a person shows weight gain it is pretty certain that he is not taking his drug in the right dose. Weight gain is truly a problem since some people take these drugs for relatively prolonged periods — for months at a time. Because of the weight gain, or because of feeling better after a few weeks on these drugs, quite often a person will start lowering the dose or stop taking the drug without consulting his physician. Since the depressed person may not have the ability to produce an adequate amount of the free-circulating norepinephrine to allow him to efficiently cope with the real problems of his everyday life, stopping the drug or lowering the dose without consulting his physician may lead to a return of the depression. Depression is the kind of condition in which the person should continue to take his drug at the prescribed dose until specifically told otherwise by his physician. We see not only the problem of taking too much of a drug but also the problem of not taking enough or not continuing to take it for the specified period of time. Indeed, a few people seem to have an inborn lack of ability to produce and release enough norepinephrine in their brains to cope with everyday life. These people may have to take a tricyclic antidepressive drug for life to correct a malfunction in the physiology of the brain. Depression is not a matter of lack of character or learning to live right. It requires the same kind of continued therapy that is needed by a person who is a diabetic, who has to take insulin to help correctly adjust his metabolizing of sugar. There is no nobility in going through life psychologically crippled when we have the ability to help correct that part of brain chemistry that will allow a person to live with efficiency and with the normal cycles of sadness and happiness. The fact that a particular chemical works in the brain, as opposed to working in the pancreas, the big toe, or anywhere else, does not make it any more morally right or wrong than any other drug. I cannot emphasize too strongly that the effect of a tricyclic antidepressant is not to make a person artificially happy but only to repair a faulty brain function. It allows the brain to function in a more normal fashion and so to prevent excessive, debilitating amounts of sadness and grief. When grief, sadness, hopelessness, loss of self-respect become so severe as to be debilitating and destructive or to prevent a person from finding constructive ways out of his problems, he needs both psychiatric and pharmacological help.

▶▶▶ NONTRICYCLIC ANTIDEPRESSANTS

Drugs other than the tricyclic antidepressive type may be used for the relief of episodic depression of a mild sort. These depressions have been called the "existential" depressions, since they are a part of everyday living for all of us. In these cases, the problem does not seem to be a failure to have an adequate amount of free norepinephrine in the brain but rather, it seems to be the need, on a temporary basis, for relief of a severe feeling of sadness or hopelessness produced by life's events.

The usual pharmacological approach to this difficulty has been to use the combination of a stimulant drug, such as amphetamine, that will cause a release of central norepinephrine as well as a blockage of its uptake, and a sedative-hypnotic, such as a barbiturate, or a tranquilizer, for example, meprobamate. This type of combination produces a stimulated, elated mood without over-agitation. One combination of this type is Dexamyl®, which contains 5 mg to 10 mg of amphetamine and 100 mg of amobarbital. Used in Britain, it is known as a "purple heart." These stimulant-sedative combinations differ in mode of action and therapeutic purpose from the tricyclic antidepressants. They do not cause the long-term stabilization and more normal state of brain function that the tricyclic drugs bring about. They do provide immediate, temporary relief in an intolerable situation. This does not mean that they are useless drugs. Indeed, when you have had the loss of a loved one, or experienced some other traumatic, grief-laden event, these drugs work immediately to help you get through a period of a few days, or a few weeks at most, in which the depression or sadness might otherwise be overwhelming. However, since both types of drugs in combinations, the amphetamines and the tranquilizers or sedatives, have a number of associated problems when used on a prolonged basis, they are used best for brief periods of therapy for dulling intense grief. Here, I make the distinction between grief, where there is a traumatic event giving a reason for sorrow, and depression, in which the sadness reaction to the life situation is excessive in degree and length and for which the tricyclic drugs are used. The latter is the case of faulty brain chemistry and the need for restoring normal brain physiology on a relatively long-term basis so that the patient can begin to cope with life again. On the other hand, the stimulant-sedative combinations are used for a sorrow that would be considered normal but so overwhelming that the patient would be better off with some degree of reduction in grief for a temporary period. It certainly would be very questionable therapy to use a stimulant-sedative combination for a prolonged period. On the other hand, a person who needs the tricyclic drugs often requires them for very long periods or for life to maintain normal brain physiology.

My own opinion on the use of these substances is that the tricyclic type antidepressants are normalizing. They return the person to a normal condition of brain chemistry. I regard this as no different from treating a broken leg, diabetes, heart trouble, or any other simple physical event. Certainly, there seems to be no more advantage in continuing to suffer from depressions due to inadequate brain chemistry than to suffer from inadequacy in the chemistry of any other organ. On the other hand, I see the use of the stimulant-sedative combinations as a temporary "crutch" to get through a bad period of life. By the term "crutch," I don't mean to imply that there is no proper use for these drugs. All of us, episodically, will suffer from physical or mental "broken legs." Not to use a "crutch" in these circumstances can be as stupid as using a "crutch" all the time when it really isn't needed. To follow the analogy further, if you use a crutch when you have a broken leg it will help restore the bone and muscle in the leg. On the other hand, if you use a crutch when your leg is perfectly well, it will cause the development of atrophy and weakness of the muscle. So I think that drugs of this nature can be used intelligently, episodically, to improve your life. To use them constantly may lead to a severe debilitation. However, as I mentioned, this is only my opinion. Others may have different, but also valid, opinions as to the appropriateness of the use of such "crutch-like" chemicals.

▶▶▶ THE TREATMENT OF MANIA

A condition closely related to depression, but that appears to be its exact opposite, is called "mania." Many people suffer not only from extreme debilitating depression but also, every few months or years, swing to the opposite pole — elated, over-happy, and frantic activity. This "elation" phase is called mania. Mania used to be suppressed with major tranquilizers like chlorpromazine. For severe mania this is still the best treatment but a very important and exciting discovery has been made with the introduction of the chemical lithium into use for the treatment of mania. Its use, in the majority of cases, can eliminate the manic upswings of the mood cycle and, sometimes, the depressive downswings. By using lithium, and sometimes with the use of tricyclic drugs as well, people who suffer from a cyclic mood disorder can live normal lives.

At this time we do not know the means by which lithium blocks the hyper-excitement and elation. There are some interesting theories but they are not well enough studied yet for us to discuss its mechanism of action.

The major problem with lithium therapy is the exceedingly low therapeutic safety ratio, almost 1:2. The dose necessary to control the elation and hyper-excitement of mania is very close to the dose that causes a toxic reaction. The toxic symptoms of lithium overdose are tremor of the hands, fatigue, muscular weakness, slurred speech, blurred vision, dizziness, and incoordination. At higher doses, it can cause convulsions and death. Therefore, it is necessary for the physician to monitor very closely the blood levels of lithium at all times during treatment to ensure that an adequate amount is taken, but one under the toxic level. This may become a bit of a chore since one often takes this chemical for prolonged periods of time, years, in order to maintain the control of the mania. Even after the patient is stabilized on lithium, many physicians will want to check his blood levels each month. Another major problem with lithium therapy is to try to convince a person who is excited, happy, and elated that he is sick. Lithium controls excessive, inappropriate elation. So, who wants to be less happy? The drug brings a person into normal rhythm of happiness-unhappiness that we all generally feel. Still, what arguments can be used to get a person who is hyper-happy to go on to this kind of therapy? It's hard to want to become more normal, even if the excessive happiness, elation, and excitement are doing great damage to a person's life situation. Too much happiness can cause as many problems as too little. Sometimes people with mania have to be involuntarily hospitalized, or else their families have to exert a lot of pressure on them to seek proper treatment.

Chapter 12

Shotgun Cold Remedies

Perhaps no single disease is so often treated with drugs as the common cold. Further, probably no disease has so many nonphysicians prescribing remedies. It is almost a national pastime to advise about colds. If you tell someone that you have a cold, he will usually say he's either just over one or has a worse one than you do. Then, he will prescribe a remedy that probably won't work. The same preoccupation with the cold occurs in mass media advertising.

A number of multiple drug compounds have been put together that are supposed to help relieve the symptoms of the common cold. These compounds are a mixture of a group of chemicals, each of which is aimed at one of the cold symptoms. A true cold is caused by one of a number of possible viruses that cause upper respiratory infections. As of now, we have no effective therapy to combat these viruses. The combination remedies will not cure a cold and may or may not be effective for any one or all of the symptoms of a cold. These mixtures or compounds are "shotguns," attempts to cover a whole area of symptoms in the hope that one or more of the chemicals can help with at least some of the disturbances. None of these compounds is advertised as a cure for a cold.

What appears to be a cold may be many different things. First, a cold may be an allergic response. Cold symptoms, considered as "colds," may be a response to some chemical in the air, or possibly, a drug or food, that causes a histamine release in the sinus areas. A second possibility is that some of the viruses responsible for colds may produce toxic substances that act as allergic agents to produce a release of histamine. In these two cases, antihistaminic therapy can be useful in relieving some of the cold symptoms.

Another aspect of the common cold is that it may not really be a cold. Many disorders, other than the viral infections causing a true common cold, have symptoms similar to those of the cold. For example, the sore throat that is often associated with a cold could really be either a primary streptococcus infection or a secondary germ infection with a viral cold also present. Although we have no antibiotics that are effective in the elimination of viruses causing colds, we have very effective antibiotics for the treatment of the more serious bacterial infections that can cause similar symptoms. If you have one of these serious infections and if you try to relieve its symptoms with a "shotgun" cold remedy, you may be covering up the signs of a type of infection that should be treated by rapid, potent antibiotic therapy. On the other hand, unless you have proof that there are germs present that are sensitive to an antibiotic, you should not take antibiotics, with all the hangups associated with their use, when you merely have some sniffles and sneezes. It is because of this potential association with more dangerous disorders that it is fair to say that the symptoms of a cold are not something to be sneezed at. Most of the time, however, the more dangerous disorders bring with them a fever of over 100 degrees, severe sore throat, chest pains or difficulty in breathing, stiff neck, a violent headache, or other symptoms not usually associated with a simple cold.

Finally, there is the case in which the cold is strictly of a viral nature. You have the symptoms of sore throat, sore muscles, congestion in the sinuses, sore eyes, weakness and fatigue, and a general debilitation. We have no means, at this time, of effectively stopping the virus that causes the cold. If the virus is one of the kind that produces toxins that cause a release of histamine or if your symptoms are caused by an allergy, you may be able to relieve some of these symptoms with an antihistamine. Fundamentally, however, you will have to live with your cold for a week or two. There really is nothing you can do about it.

▶▶▶ COMPONENTS OF COLD MEDICINES

A primary component of a "shotgun" cold remedy you might use would be an analgesic — aspirin, acetaminophen, or phenacetin. This is taken to relieve body aches and pains, headache, or a sore throat. Aspirin is a very good pain-reducing drug for these sorts of things. Second, the compound will generally contain an antihistamine, in case you don't really have a virus infection but are responding to an allergic state, or in case you do have a virus and it is producing an antigen that causes the release of histamine and therefore an allergic response, particularly mucous congestion. Third, quite often, shotgun compounds will contain one of the belladonnas already discussed, atropine, hyoscyamine, or scopolamine, in the hope that the drying effect on mucous tissue will help stop dripping. However, as was mentioned earlier, the dose of belladonna necessary to get an antisecretory effect, that is, to stop the dripping in the nose and sinuses, is such that it will cause dryness in the mouth, ringing in the ears, and a rapid heartbeat. The side effects may become quite unpleasant at this high dose. Because of these side effects, the amounts of belladonnas used in the "shotgun" cold remedies are usually so low as to be essentially ineffective. Fourth, the "shotguns" usually contain a decongestant of the ephedrine class. I have not yet discussed this type of drug. Finally, the compounds often contain vitamin C. Large doses of vitamin C have been proposed by some authorities for the prevention of colds, but it is still a very controversial subject. We won't discuss vitamin C at this time, since there is a chapter on vitamins. See Chapter 6 for the belladonnas and Chapter 7 for the discussion of analgesics.

Antihistamines

Histamine is an interesting chemical. It was discovered in 1906, and in 1910 extensive studies were carried out by Henry Dale. From these studies we have learned much about what histamine does in the body. Yet, we have really no good idea of what benefit it is for the body. It is hard to believe that a chemical as prevalent in the body and as pharmacologically active on all sorts of tissues isn't there for a particular reason. But the fact of the matter is, we are not at all sure what that reason is. For the most part, the best single explanation of the presence of histamine, and this only accounts for a part of its various actions, is its usefulness in situations of infection. It causes an expansion of very small blood vessels and a release of some of the fluids from these small vessels into the surrounding tissue. When there is an infection it is necessary to quickly get lots of white blood cells to that area, so that they may seal off and destroy the germs that are causing the infection. Certainly the best way to do this is to cause a rapid increase in blood flow and a slight opening up of the blood vessels to let more cells and fluid seep out of the blood. This is what histamine does. Further, histamine is located in cells that are found throughout the body. Thus, it is easily available, all over the body, to help with the appropriate kind of response to an infection. Whether this is its main function is difficult to say. But it is at least one possible explanation for the presence of histamine in our bodies.

This increase in the size of the small blood vessels and letting of fluid out of the blood vessels into surrounding tissue is what causes the triple response to histamine that I described in Chapter 2: itch, flare, and wheal. When the area starts to itch, you scratch it. The scratching causes the flare. The flare occurs because of the expansion of the blood vessels. Vessels become bigger and red, causing the associated skin area to look red. Finally, since there is a release of fluids from the blood vessels and an expansion of the blood vessels in the area, the skin begins to puff up. This puffing is the histamine wheal.

This same reaction takes place in mucous membranes. When it happens in mucous membrane, instead of causing the itch, flare, wheal phenomenon, it mainly causes the vessels in the mucous membrane to swell and to release fluid into the mucous tissue from blood vessels. This is what clogs up the cold sufferer. It is the swelling of mucosal tissue, due to the enlargement of the blood vessels and the infiltration of fluid from the blood vessels into the tissues, that causes congestion and a runny nose. If the same kind of histamine release takes place farther down toward the lungs, then there will be a swelling of the tissue in the breathing tubes, the bronchi. So, the congestion in your sinuses and nose found with a cold or hay-fever-type reaction is due to a histamine reaction in this area. This swelling, plus a constriction of the muscles surrounding the bronchi, is what produces bronchial asthma. The same kind of histamine response of the swelling of the blood vessels and release of fluids into tissue in the arm, leg, or other skin area will cause the triple response of itch, flare, and wheal.

Antihistamine Action

Antibodies are chemicals formed in your body in response to allergy-causing chemicals called antigens, which come from your environment — air, food, drugs, and so on. Antibodies cause the release of histamine. On the surfaces of the histamine reacting organs are places called "receptors." If histamine molecules occupy these "receptors," the organ will respond. Antihistamines act by going to "receptor" sites on the surfaces of the cells that react to histamine.

They block the occupation of these sites by histamine. They compete with histamine for the site. When an antihistamine is on the receptor site, it just lies there passively and does not cause the reaction. This blocks the receptor site, preventing histamine from being able to get into it. As long as the antihistamine molecule is on the receptor site the histamine cannot act. For this reason, in an allergic response to mechanical pressure, pollen, chemicals, foods, in many kinds of bronchial asthma, and in cold symptoms produced by viruses that produce an antigen that causes a histamine release, there will be a dramatic and rapid reduction of symptoms with the use of an antihistamine. Indeed, within as little as five to about forty-eight hours you may expect to see the symptoms go away because the histamine can no longer act. On the other hand, if the congestion and swelling are not caused by histamine release, you can take an antihistamine from now until doomsday and it isn't going to do you any good. So, results from using an antihistamine will depend upon whether you are lucky enough to hit the source of the problem. You may or may not. It's hard to know ahead of time.

Antihistamine Drugs

The correct dose of an antihistamine varies between 2 mg and 100 mg per tablet, depending on the particular antihistamine you are using.

A few of the common antihistamines are diphenhydramine (Benadryl), carbinoxamine (Clistin), tripelennamine (Pyribenzamine), pyrilamine (Neo-Antergan, Copsamine, Paraminyl, Thylogen), antazoline (Antistine), methapyrilene (Dozar, Histadyl, Buffadyne, Thenylene), cyproheptadine (Periactin), chlorpheniramine (Chlor-Trimeton, Teldrin, Antagonate, Histaspan), dexbrompheniramine (Dimetane, Disomer), dexchlorpheniramine (Polaramine), chlorcyclizine (Fedrazil), triprolidine (Actidil), and promethazine (Phenergan). There is another group of antihistamines that have the very different property of protecting against motion sickness. This is not related to their antihistaminic effect.

These are dimenhydrinate (Dramamine), cyclizine (Marezine), and meclizine (Bonine). These are discussed in the chapter on stomach drugs.

The antihistamines are highly effective for the relief of allergic conditions. Within five to forty-eight hours the symptoms of most allergies will be nearly eliminated. On the other hand, these drugs do have some unpleasant side effects. Approximately half of all people who take them will have some degree of undesired side effects, even when taken at an appropriate dose. Luckily, the side effects of a given drug tend to be specific for a particular individual and not associated with the antihistaminic properties of that drug. This means that if you are taking an antihistamine and you have unpleasant side effects, try a different antihistamine. It may be equally effective in giving protection againt histamine action but will have fewer side effects for you. The side effects are somewhat dose related. The more drug that you take, the more likely you are to get the side effects. It is not uncommon while under antihista-minic therapy to try two or three different antihistamines at differ-ent doses to get the ideal drug that gives the maximum antihista-minic relief and, at the same time, the fewest possible side effects.

The first, and most common, of the side effects with these drugs is sedation. It is an unpleasant form of sedation, not like that of the sedative-hypnotics, but a more "blah," droopy, and drowsy feeling. It is like the feeling of sleepiness that comes with tranquilizers of the phenothiazine type, such as chlorpromazine. Indeed, these an-tihistamines are closely related to the phenothiazine drugs. This sleepiness occurs in most people. However, choosing the right anti-histamine can reduce the severity of this problem. The sedation from histamines combines with alcohol and other hypnotics to produce an even greater effect. You must be very careful if you drink or take sleeping pills while on antihistamine therapy. Other, less common side effects can occur with these drugs. They are muscular weak-ness, fatigue, headache, dry mouth, nervousness, vomiting, stomach distress, low blood pressure, tightness in the chest, tingling of the hands, and dizziness. Although this list sounds ominous, these side effects, when they occur, are usually not too severe. Also, you can get around them if you find just the right dose of the right antihistamine. So you can get a good antihistamine effect and, at the same time, a minimum of side effects.

Antihistamines are the drugs of choice to treat a drug-caused allergy. Yet, they, themselves, can on occasion produce an allergic response, that is, cause a histamine release. Luckily, this is a rare reaction to antihistamine drugs.

Antihistamines are often regarded as very benign compounds and are sometimes casually left lying around the house. This is a mistake. Antihistamines are too often coming to be the cause of accidental poisoning or used in suicides. Their therapeutic safety ratio is quite good. It takes at least fifty to one hundred tablets to kill an adult, but children are quite sensitive to these compounds. They can die from as few as twenty to thirty tablets. The symptoms of toxic poisoning with the antihistamines are excitement, hallucinations, incoordination, convulsions, large, dilated pupils, flushed face, and fever. A child can go into a deep coma and be dead within two to eighteen hours. A word of warning, antihistamines are not benign drugs. They must be treated with the same precautions and care that one uses with other drugs.

Ephedrine Decongestants

A common ingredient in the shotgun remedies for colds that we have not yet discussed are decongestants of the ephedrine type. Ephedrine is one of the oldest drugs known to man. It had been used in China, in an herb, for over five thousand years before it was introduced into Western medicine. It was used to promote stimulation of the central nervous system, to cause strengthening of the heart, and to decongest by causing shrinkage of the blood vessels in the mucous areas of the nose and sinuses.

Ephedrine, chemically, is closely related to amphetamine and cocaine. All of the ephedrine-like drugs are very similar chemically to the cocaine-amphetamine type. However, they differ in a very important way from cocaine and amphetamines. Whereas cocaine and amphetamines are taken predominantly for effects on the brain and go into the brain with great ease, chemicals of the ephedrine class are very badly absorbed by the brain and act on the rest of the body, with little central stimulating effect. With some of them, such as ephedrine, there is some degree of stimulating effect on the brain, but it is minimal. For others of this same series, there is no stimulating effect on the brain.

The decongestant action of these chemicals is produced by making the small blood vessels in the nose, sinuses, and other areas constrict — just the opposite of what histamine does. The drugs do this by directly stimulating points on the smooth muscles that surround these small blood vessels. They mimic the natural, body hormone epinephrine. When these smooth muscles surrounding the small blood vessels in the mucous areas get tighter, they constrict the vessels. This causes a shrinkage of the tissue that has been engorged with blood and has been secreting extra fluids that seep out of the blood vessels.

The drugs of this type that you are likely to run into can be in two forms. You may either take them orally in a pill, or you can squirt them straight onto tissue as a drop or spray. Drugs that you will quite commonly see used as decongestants are phenylephrine (Neo-Synephrine, Isophrin), hydroxyamphetamine (Paredrine), naphazoline (Privine), tetrahydrozoline (Tyzine), oxymetazoline (Afrin), xylometazoline (Otrivin), cyclopentamine (Clopane), phenylpropanolamine;° in the form of nasal inhalants, you might find propylhexedrine (Benzedrex) or tuaminoheptane (Tuamine). You'll note in this list that there are drugs that have also been recommended for use in the eye. For example, tetrahydrozoline is found in some of the newer eyedrops to make redness go away. In

---

° Phenylpropanolamine is also a standard ingredient in diet aids. It seems to temporarily reduce appetite due to its side effect of drying the mouth and reducing stomach activity. It is usually combined with a cellulose product that produces a nondigestible bulk in the stomach.

this case, the drug is acting by the same mechanism as when used for a nasal spray. It causes a constriction of the small blood vessels that are making your eyes red and watery just as it causes the blood vessels in your nose to constrict to make your nose less watery. Please be careful, however, never to put anything in your eyes unless the drug is specifically designed for use in the eyes. Your eyes are very sensitive to chemicals and could be severely harmed by improper use of drugs.

Problems Associated with Decongestant Use

All of the decongestants of the ephedrine class have one great common disadvantage. They can cause an "after congestion." They can even produce chronic congestion if used for a long time. This is to say, if you use one of these compounds in your nose, it will provide relief for a period, but then there is rebound. The rebound congestion can make the problem worse. If you keep using nasal decongestants over a number of days, the nasal decongestant itself will start to cause the congestion that you are trying to fight. Further, the constricting power of these decongestants is rapidly tolerated. This means that their effectiveness as decongestants goes away, more and more, every time you take a dose. Tolerance can develop in a few days with persistent use. So here is the problem. You want to decongest yourself so that you can breathe more easily. However, if you take these drugs too often, as often as a few times a day, and you take them for too long, over a few days, instead of producing a nice long decongestion, the length of the decongesting action becomes shorter and shorter and, then, the drugs start to cause a rebound congestion that can become chronic, that is, you will always have a runny nose. This is a wicked cycle. In an attempt to obtain relief, you may cause the problem to get worse. More people than you would believe have become tolerant to, have a chronic congestion from, and are now psychologically and physiologically dependent upon the use of decongestants, taking them either orally or directly into the nose. The same principle applies to the effects of these drugs when they are placed in the eye. Initially, you may have an effective clearing of your eyes with the use of tetrahydrozoline. But this effect becomes tolerated relatively rapidly and, indeed, there can be a rebound of redness. This discussion is not meant to discourage you from using decongestants to feel better. On the other hand, you should be aware that if you use them too often they will lose their ability to help and may cause a serious problem.

▶▶▶ THE TREATMENT OF THE COMMON COLD

For the most part, people either believe in a cold remedy or they don't. Perhaps belief is the strongest element present in any of the cold remedies. The doses of the drugs in shotgun remedies tend to be quite low — usually too low to get any sensible therapeutic effect. There are problems associated with the use of these drugs — they either lose their efficacy due to tolerance or they produce unpleasant side effects. On the other hand, if a cold causes you to ache and hurt, certainly aspirin is a good drug. It is relatively safe and can aid your comfort by relieving sore muscles or any other kind of body soreness and pain. The dose of the belladonnas in the shotguns is probably too little to do any good, unless you take a large dose that would cause rapid heartbeat and other unpleasant side effects. The decongestant can help for a little while, but if you take too much, for too long, it will cause more problems than you already have. The use of the antihistamines is fine, if you happen to have an allergic response causing your symptoms. Whether you do or not will be determined, I suppose, after the fact. You will get benefit from antihistamines if there is an allergic response or you won't if there is no allergic response. And finally, the use of vitamins in such mixtures is probably useless. So, on the whole, when you are taking a shotgun cold remedy, be aware that: (1) you're not curing a cold, (2) the odds are you're not going to get a great deal of help from it, and (3) it helps a lot to believe in a particular cold remedy you're taking. The biggest single effect of these medications is the so-called "placebo" effect. The more you expect the medicine to help, the more it can make you feel better.

Quite often there is one final drug that is added to these mixtures. This is caffeine, usually in the dose of 150 mg, the same amount that is in a cup of coffee. Perhaps if the effects of the antihistamines make you sleepy, caffeine provides stimulation. There seems to be no other reasonable therapeutic rationale for taking caffeine when you have a cold.

▷ Chapter 13

Vitamins and Minerals

Perhaps no single class of drugs is so misused in our country, so much a target of misunderstanding, misrepresentation and downright quackery as vitamins and minerals. Fortunately, for most people, the misuse of vitamins and minerals usually results only in an unnecessary expenditure of funds. However, in some cases, the excessive vitamin and mineral supplementation can lead to harm.

There is little question that the average healthy adult who has an adequate diet and is paying appropriate attention to the mixtures of different types of foods that are good for him does not need to waste his money by adding supplementary vitamins and minerals to his diet. These drugs don't give a person "super health." Further, there is not yet any uncontested evidence that any of the vitamins or minerals can prevent the occurrence of any disease other than the particular disease associated with a deficiency of specific vitamins or minerals. In other words, the only proven benefits of these drugs is their use as supplements to the diet when it has been shown to be deficient due to a particular faddism in the use of foods, lack of attention in obtaining an adequately balanced diet, or because of a disorder that causes an excessive body use of a specific vitamin or mineral. Only in these cases is there any need to have dietary supplementation at all. The majority of people who take these compounds are wasting their money and, in some cases, harming themselves. They probably won't obtain more energy, better looks, resistance to disease or any other benefit by taking them.

There are two basic types of vitamins, water-soluble and fat-soluble. The water-soluble vitamins include B-complex vitamins, vitamin C, and the flavonoids. The fat-soluble vitamins are vitamins A, D, H, K, and E. The water-soluble vitamins are not harmful if they are taken in excessive doses. The body will rid itself of unnecessary amounts of the water-soluble vitamins. On the other hand, some of the fat-soluble vitamins can cause serious toxic reactions if they are taken in excessive amounts, since they accumulate in your body beyond your requirements.

▶▶▶ WATER-SOLUBLE VITAMINS

Vitamin B_1 (Thiamine)

Thiamine was the first vitamin of the B-complex to be identified. It was first found by Funk, who coined the term "Vitamin" to indicate that this particular type of chemical was vital for life. It was discovered in a search for a compound that would overcome the disease beriberi. Beriberi had first been identified in Java after the natives had switched from eating unpolished rice to polished rice as a major part of their diet. It was later found that the outside husk of rice is rich in vitamin B_1, so eating highly polished rice deprived people of this necessary vitamin.

Thiamine is practically devoid of any side effects if it is taken in appropriate amounts. There have been a few cases reported of toxic reactions but these are probably rare hypersensitivities to the vitamin. Thiamine acts to help regulate the burning of foods in your body. Thus, the amount of thiamine that you need is a function of the number of calories you consume in food. Thiamine is a relatively common ingredient of most foods, particularly meat and other proteinaceous foods. The daily recommended thiamine dose is 0.5 mg per thousand calories eaten. Generally, the maximum absorbed oral dose is between 8 mg and 15 mg a day. We burn, on the average, about 1 mg of thiamine per day.*

In our country we seldom see the severe form of beriberi, but occasionally in some people, a mild thiamine deficiency can develop if they try to live on a diet that is totally lacking in thiamine. This is not a very easy disorder to get. The signs of thiamine deficiency are the symptoms of beriberi. Its first symptoms are loss of appetite, muscular weakness, pain, a tingling sensation in fingers and toes, and a low body temperature. If the disorder becomes severe, there can be major changes in muscle strength, and paralysis will set in. Also, there are severe effects on the heart.

Very little thiamine is stored in the body. Because of this small storage pool, you have to ingest it regularly. Your average thiamine intake should be adequate for every ten-day period. You don't have to have enough every day but you should have enough every ten days. This differs from most vitamins that have relatively large stores in the body. You can be depleted of thiamine in as little as ten days if there is none in your diet, whereas for most vitamins, the depletion time is many months. Again, the only known therapeutic utility of thiamine is for people who have thiamine deficiencies. If you obtain amounts in excess of your needs, your body discards it.

* The term "Required Daily Allowance" (RDA) is the amount of each vitamin and mineral that a government commission has determined to be necessary. It is now the common expression for appropriate dose.

B₂ (Riboflavin)

Riboflavin, or vitamin B_2, is also found in many meat and proteinaceous substances. It, as does thiamine, acts to regulate the energy producing processes of your body.

At its normal doses, it has no obvious effects upon the body, and toxicity from this vitamin is unknown. The body will eliminate any excess amount of riboflavin beyond the amount it needs. The recommended intake of riboflavin per day is 0.3 mg per 1,000 calories of food.

Symptoms of riboflavin deficiency are sores and eruptions, particularly found in the corners of the mouth and of other mucous areas such as in the nose or the throat. If you were placed on a diet totally riboflavin free, it would take you about three or more months to develop these symptoms. The normal body stores of riboflavin seem to be adequate to maintain you for at least three months. Again, the only therapeutic use established for riboflavin is for people who have a riboflavin deficiency in their diet.

Nicotinic Acid (Niacin, Nicotinamide)

First, nicotinic acid should be distinguished from nicotine. These are two very different drugs. For this reason I shall use the term niacin, or nicotinamide, rather than nicotinic acid.

Niacin acts to help the body regulate its energy producing sources. Its only known therapeutic use is to overcome the symptoms of the disease pellagra, which is caused by a deficiency of this vitamin. The chief symptoms of pellagra in its subclinical, or non-severe, form are headaches, dizziness, insomnia, depression, impairment of memory, and in certain cases, hallucinations and psychosis. In addition to these symptoms, severe pellagra can cause considerable digestive tract troubles with soreness and diarrhea. The tongue may become red and swollen with sores on it. Its most distinguishing characteristic is the eruption of reddish spots on the backs of the hands that look something like sunburn. Later on, other areas such as the forehead, neck, and feet can be involved in this sunburn-like eruption.

The recommended dosage of niacin is 6.6 mg per 1,000 calories per day. Toxic reactions to niacin are possible, but in experimental dogs one has to give a dose of over 4 gm or 5 gm a day to cause any trouble. Human deaths have not occurred so far.

Pyridoxine (Vitamin B_6)

Pyridoxine is involved with the orderly burning of the protein foods in the body. Its deficiency will cause an incorrect balance in the use of this energy source. The symptoms of a deficiency of pyridoxine are sores in the eyes, nose, and mouth. This can be produced within as little as a few weeks of a diet that is lacking in vitamin B_6. The storage pool of vitamin B_6 is larger than for B_1 but smaller than for riboflavin. If there is a continuation of a deficiency of B_6, the symptoms are convulsions and a general overactivity of the central nervous system. Taking the drug isoniazid for tuberculosis causes a rapid metabolism of B_6. Often a person on isoniazid therapy is given a B_6 supplement.

The requirement for an adult is 2.0 mg per day of B_6, if you have an intake of 100 grams of protein per day. Since this particular vitamin regulates protein utilization, its intake level is related to the amount of protein eaten per day. There is little evidence that, in the average person, toxic effects of pyridoxine can occur even with large overdoses.

Ascorbic Acid (Vitamin C)

Vitamin C has had an interesting history. Some people have claimed it protects against the common cold, heart trouble, and most of the other ills of mankind. Many of these claims are interesting. However, as of now, it is fair to say that there is no documented evidence, that is, without controversy, that vitamin C (ascorbic acid) is beneficial for the treatment or prevention of any condition except scurvy, the disease that results from a deficiency of vitamin C. Possibly, studies in the future may show vitamin C to have benefits for man other than the prevention of scurvy, but at this time, the evidence is too cloudy for us to make any very positive statement one way or the other.

The major function of vitamin C is to aid in the maintenance of the connective tissues of the body such as ligaments, tendons, etc. Therefore, when there is an inadequate amount of vitamin C in the body, these connective tissues, which hold the cells apart, begin to break down. Small pinpoints of bleeding will appear under the skin as small red spots, all over the body, including the eye. However, prior to this, there are mood changes in people suffering from scurvy. They become very mean, irritable, and argumentative. In the final stages of scurvy, a person's legs become so weak that he has to be helped to walk.

To make a person deficient in vitamin C is not easy unless you set about it rather deliberately. Scurvy was first found on the British sailing ships, in the old days. It was a prevalent condition when people were on voyages for a long period of time eating only jerky, salt pork, and hardtack. However, James Lind showed that by taking fresh citrus fruits, such as limes, on board the ship, scurvy could be prevented. The British sailors picked up the nickname "Limeys" because of their use of this citrus fruit as a source of vitamin C to protect against scurvy.

Vitamin C deficiency, or scurvy, still does occur occasionally in the United States. I know one case that occurred in a small town to a man who had bought a bar. He was trying to save all of his money by attempting to live on a diet of pretzels and beer. In approximately seven months' time he came down with the classic scurvy symptoms. However, since it does take many months of a diet completely lacking in vitamin C before the body pool is exhausted, this is not an easy disorder to get. The recommended daily dose of vitamin C is 40 mg to 60 mg. Vitamin C content is very high in all orange, lemon, and lime juices. This allows people who require vitamin C therapy to use the same technique that Lind did, that is, to get their full vitamin replacement by drinking fruit juices. However, many other foods besides these also have high levels of vitamin C. There are no known toxic effects even from very high doses of vitamin C. The body seems to just throw off what it does not need.

Recently, studies have indicated that doses of 2 gm to 10 gm of vitamin C taken for at least a week prior to the onset of a cold will reduce the runny nose, coughing, and unpleasant feeling associated with the disease. There is no evidence to suggest that the viral infection that causes a cold is blocked. However, the symptom reduction is a worthwhile effect of this vitamin.

Flavonoids (Vitamin P)

Flavonoids (vitamin P) are presently available as three different drugs, Rutin, Quercetin, and Hesperidin. They are occasionally used to try to keep fluid from leaking out of the blood vessels causing bruise-like spots under the skin. However, this has not been proven as a necessary or effective therapy. Indeed, there is little evidence, at the present time, that the flavonoids have any particular important physiological function, or even whether they should be characterized as vitamins. Further, there are no specific deficiency symptoms that have ever been related to them and, at present, there is no evidence that they are essential to man.

Other Water-soluble Vitamins

There are some other water-soluble vitamins that are presently recommended. For example, pantothenic acid in daily doses of 5 mg to 10 mg and biotin at a daily intake of 150 mcg to 300 mcg. However, the reason for the use of these substances is not well worked out. We don't even know for sure if they are really necessary for health.

▶▶▶ FAT-SOLUBLE VITAMINS

Vitamin A (Retinol)

Vitamin A has a number of important roles in the body but perhaps the most direct one is in the retina of the eye. With a deficiency of vitamin A, the first symptom that will be noticed is an interference of the ability of the person to see in dim light. This disorder is called night blindness. However, it takes a number of months before night blindness can be induced even with a diet totally deficient of vitamin A. Therefore, we know the body pools of this vitamin are rather large. If a vitamin A deficiency continues for up to seven to nine months, there will be problems with drying of the skin and eruptions. There will be impairment of the retinal cells that can ultimately lead to blindness if one has a total lack of vitamin A in his diet long enough. An increased number of kidney stones have been found in humans who have been deprived of vitamin A as well as changes in the gastrointestinal tract that cause diarrhea. However, as was mentioned, it takes months of a total depletion of vitamin A to cause these problems.

The recommended human dose is approximately 5,000 units of vitamin A per day. Vitamin A is found in butter, egg yolk, and, particularly, in cod liver oil. An even more potent source of vitamin A is percomorph liver oil. You should be very careful to distinguish between percomorph liver oil and the far less potent cod liver oil when considering sources of this vitamin.

An excess of vitamin A can kill. Children are particularly sensitive to this vitamin. A toxic dose for children is between 50,000 and 500,000 units a day. Adults also have died from overdoses of vitamin A. One of the worst problems associated with taking this vitamin is the six month or more buildup of an excessive dosage before the first appearance of the clinical signs of poisoning. If you are taking too much vitamin A, it may be six months before you know that you're being poisoned by it.

The earliest signs of vitamin A poisoning are irritability, loss of appetite, and itching. This is followed by fatigue, loss of body hair, and enlargement of the lymph nodes. Finally, brain tumors can develop from a consistent overdose of this vitamin. An interesting, but unusual, example of acute poisoning by vitamin A has been found in a man eating polar bear liver. The polar bear's liver is a particularly high source of vitamin A, containing up to 35,000 units of vitamin A per gm. Symptoms of sluggishness, irritability, irresistible desire to sleep, severe headache and vomiting, and then, finally, a generalized peeling of the skin can occur in as little as twenty-four hours after eating polar bear liver.

Vitamin D (Ergosterol, Calciferol, Dihydrocholesterol)

Vitamin D has been called the sunshine vitamin. It was first discovered by noticing that urban children, particularly in the North Temperate Zone, often developed rickets, whereas children who wore fewer clothes, ran around outside in tropical areas, were exposed to a more intense sunlight did not get rickets. Some thought that this disease was due to a lack of fresh air and sunshine. Others claimed that it was a dietary deficiency. Actually it turned out that both were right. Vitamin D is obtained from many animal sources. It is found in milk, fish oils, and other proteinaceous foods. It is also formed in the skin of a person who is exposed to sunlight. Your own skin manufactures it when you are out in the sun.

Following the discovery of the relationship between the development of rickets by children in urban areas and a deficiency of vitamin D, a massive program was begun in the United States in the 1930s to overcome this deficiency by enriching many foods such as milk, bread, and others, with vitamin D. It was at this time that the general public first became aware of the existence of vitamins. A great many of the present beliefs held by many people about the need for vitamins grew up in this era of enthusiastic propaganda. The program for the prevention of rickets by supplementing foods with vitamin D was the cause of the "oversell" of vitamin therapy. Lately, a rather different approach has been taken in considering the use of vitamin supplements. We have found that too many people are beginning to get too much vitamin D. This is one of the vitamins that can cause poisoning if too much is taken. A large number of supplemented foods are available, although you probably don't even notice that many of the foods you buy are labeled "enriched," or "vitamin D supplemented." Further, if you are in the southern part of the United States where the rays of the sun are more intense, your skin makes large amounts of vitamin D. Finally, if you take vitamin pills, in addition to these other sources, you could be harming yourself by having an overdose of vitamin D. For this reason the government is encouraging many of the manufacturers who have been supplementing their foods with vitamin D to reduce the amount of the vitamin. It is hoped that this will help to reduce the number of vitamin D toxicities that occur each year.

The major effect of vitamin D is to cause your body to produce more of a particular protein that is found in your gastrointestinal tract. This specific protein acts to bind calcium in your gastrointestinal tract. Calcium is a mineral that is very badly absorbed from the stomach and the gut, so it must be transported from the stomach and gut into the bloodstream by being bound to a specific protein. Therefore, if you don't have an adequate quantity of vitamin D you cannot obtain benefit from the calcium in the foods that you eat. It is not absorbed. For health, it is necessary to have the right amount of calcium in your system. Vitamin D helps you get this needed calcium. See the section on minerals for a discussion of calcium.

On the other hand, if you have too much vitamin D it causes an over-production of the protein that binds calcium and too much calcium is transported into your system. Therefore, the symptoms of toxicity to vitamin D are those of having too much calcium in your body. It has been found that approximately 150,000 units or more daily intake of vitamin D, for a person who has a normal sensitivity to it, may result in poisoning if continued over a long period of time. The initial signs of poisoning are: weakness, fatigue, headache, nausea, vomiting, diarrhea, problems with the kidneys causing excessive production of urine, an inability to control urine flow at night and, finally, changes in the composition of the blood. It should be pointed out that adults are not too susceptible to problems with the high level of calcium associated with vitamin D overdose. Children, however, are particularly sensitive to this disorder. In some instances, as little as 1,800 units of vitamin D per day can lead to poisoning.

The recommended dose of vitamin D varies between 400 units and 2,000 units depending upon age, whether pregnancy exists, what part of the country you live in, and other factors. The easiest way to obtain vitamin D is to take cod liver oil, though it is present in some other foods. The diet of the average person, with the various supplementations that are presently found in most foods, is fully adequate to provide plenty of vitamin D, maybe even too much.

Vitamin E (Alpha-Tocopherol)

Few vitamins have received such intensive investigation and so much publicity for so little cause as vitamin E. It was first found in wheat germ oil. This vitamin was discovered when it was found that certain animal species lower than man could not normally reproduce without its presence. This sterility was caused in the female by aborting the fetus and in the male animal by various abnormalities in the testicles. From this limited information, vitamin E has obtained the reputation of being the antisterility vitamin. Here I want to make clear the difference between sterility and potency. Sterility is the inability to have offspring. Potency, on the other hand, refers to the ability to have sexual intercourse. Vitamin E has never been shown to have anything whatsoever to do with potency. It does not affect sexual performance, nor has there been any suggestion in any animal that it might. Its only effects were shown to be in terms of the actual production of offspring by animals. Further, even in very long-term studies in which body depletion of vitamin E was total, its lack did not lead to any identifiable disease or even sterility in humans. There is a serious question whether vitamin E is a necessary vitamin in man. However, just to be on the safe side, there is a recommendation that about 25 to 30 units be taken in daily; this is not an informed recommendation. We really don't know that vitamin E has anything to do with human health. Vitamin E in even massive doses has no particular effect on man, fortunately. It is not toxic even if taken at a high dose level for a long period of time.

Other Fat-soluble Vitamins and Vitamin-like Substances

There are other vitamins, such as vitamin K and vitamin H, and other substances that are somewhat like vitamins. They are sometimes found in vitamin preparations. Examples of these vitamin-like chemicals are choline, inositol, and para-aminobenzoic acid. There is no proof of the necessity of any of these as a dietary supplement. It is very difficult to avoid getting enough of most of these possible vitamins since only minute traces, if any at all, are needed. They are very common in most foods.

▶▶▶ THE MINERALS

Calcium

Calcium is the fifth most abundant chemical element in your body. Ninety percent of it is in the skeleton but the other 10 percent is intimately involved and necessary for the appropriate functioning of every cell in your body. Further, since the body cannot manufacture calcium, it must be ingested on a reasonably regular basis. The major sources of calcium are milk and various milk products. However, other foods also contain some calcium.

As was mentioned previously in discussing vitamin D, it is not only important to have adequate calcium intake in your diet but also, there must be the right amount of vitamin D in your body, so that the calcium can be absorbed from the gut. Without the presence of the active transport of protein-bound calcium from the gut into the bloodstream, the calcium that you eat doesn't do you any good. Dietary calcium requirement varies between 200 mg and 1,500 mg a day depending upon a person's age, rate of growth, physiological state, and other factors.

The major sign of too low a calcium level in the body is weakening of the bones. The calcium in your bones and the calcium in the rest of your body are always in balance. However, the rest of your body is the preferred place for calcium. So, if you're low in calcium in your various body cells, it will be extracted from your bones to make up the deficit. It is this problem, which characterizes the disease of rickets, that affects a young, growing child, who needs about 1,200 mg of calcium a day to build new bone. If the child does not have enough calcium, both to fulfill the needs of the body and the growing bones, the bones will grow with an inadequate amount of calcium in them. They will become soft, misshapen and produce the deformities of the limbs that are characteristic of rickets. The same sort of situation can happen in an adult. There can be weakening and softening of the bones if there is either an inadequate calcium intake or an inadequate amount of vitamin D present so that calcium cannot be absorbed. However, an adult, since he is not growing at a rapid rate, does not have as high a requirement for calcium. As I mentioned, for a growing child, about 1,200 mg a day of calcium is needed; for an adult, perhaps 800 mg a day would be adequate. During pregnancy, because of the formation of bones in the fetus, an increased amount of calcium is required, between 1,200 mg and 1,500 mg of calcium per day for the mother. This is taken to ensure that there will be an adequate supply of calcium for both the mother and the baby.

Calcium is obtainable in many forms; perhaps the commonest and cheapest is calcium chloride. Either this form, or calcium carbonate, calcium lactate, calcium phosphate, or calcium resinate, can be easily absorbed by the body. Generally, it is taken with milk. Taking it with milk helps since milk has a high level of calcium itself. With two or three pints of milk a day, even a woman who is pregnant can get an adequate amount of calcium to fulfill her requirement without further supplementation.

Too much calcium in the system causes poisoning. Again, if you have too much vitamin D so that too much calcium is absorbed, or if you eat too much calcium, this can lead to a problem of too high a level of calcium in your bloodstream. The problem of a long-term excess of calcium is the formation of kidney stones. The short-term problems with very high doses of calcium are the same as for an excess of vitamin D, since, indeed, this is the same situation. The symptoms are weakness, fatigue, headache, vomiting, diarrhea, and excessive urination.

Iron

The use of iron for the treatment of pallor and weakness, particularly that associated with wounded soldiers, is very old. In ancient Hindu medicine, sheets of iron were roasted, than powdered, mixed with oil, vinegar, cow's urine, and milk to be given to warriors who had lost a lot of blood. The Greeks also used this remedy for wounded warriors. Since iron was the metal of the God of War, Mars, it was a particularly favored therapy. Iron was also believed to give greater strength to warriors. They were given drinking water in which old swords had been allowed to rust. Throughout history people have recognized that there was somehow a relationship between weakness and pallor, particularly that associated with blood loss, and a restorative property of iron or its salts.

Iron acts in the body almost entirely by forming with protein to create a complex molecule called hemoglobin. "Hemo" comes from the Greek word for blood; "-globin" is short for "globulin," a type of protein. Hemoglobin is found in the red blood cells of the body. It is this molecule that allows oxygen to be picked up in the lungs for distribution to the rest of the body. If you have an iron deficiency anemia it will be shown in the production of too few and misformed red blood cells. The result of this lack of properly formed red blood cells is the inability of the blood to carry an adequate amount of oxygen to the tissues. You might think of it as a very slow, chronic suffocation of your tissues. Since the malformation of the red blood cells in iron deficiency anemia is rather obvious, this is a very easy disease to diagnose. A trained person can look at a drop of blood under a microscope to see if there are misformed red blood cells. That is all it takes to establish whether you do or do not have an iron deficiency anemia. Another way of determining whether you have an adequate quantity of red blood cells being formed is to take a couple of drops of blood, place them in a very fine tube and spin it very, very rapidly on a centrifuge. In this way the liquid, or plasma portion of the blood, separates out and the solid portion, which is predominantly made up of red blood cells, is left. Then, by measuring on a chart, the proportion of liquid to the amount of solid in the blood can be seen. This can give evidence of the adequacy of the amount or number of red blood cells. This test takes about three to five minutes. There is no reason for anyone to assume that he either does or does not have an iron deficiency anemia because it is easily and quickly tested.

The only reason a person should have iron added to his diet is if he has a proven case of iron deficiency anemia. This is the only thing that iron is ever good for. It seems to make sense that you should take the few minutes necessary to be tested before you start taking an iron supplement. The symptoms of iron deficiency —

weakness, pallor, sometimes irritability — are the symptoms of almost every other disease known to man. So, it may be that you are suffering from something else, and if this is so and you start taking iron, you may get sicker.

There is almost no reason for an adult to develop iron deficiency anemia, except for the loss of blood. Thus, the odds are that a male will never have an iron deficiency anemia, unless he is cut or in some other way suffers a large blood loss. The body conserves iron very carefully, and there is probably plenty of iron in his food to make up for any losses. The same is true of a post-menopausal female who no longer has a loss of blood on a monthly cycle. Her iron requirements are the same as the male's, and it is also unlikely that she will develop an iron deficiency anemia.

The only population that seems to be in much risk of developing an iron deficiency anemia are females who are menstruating. For these women there is enough blood loss each month so that an iron deficiency anemia can develop. Indeed, the average American diet provides about 6 mg of iron per 1,000 calories. This is a borderline amount of iron intake for teenage girls, women, infants, and pregnant women, considering the amount of iron that is lost in growing and bleeding. The requirement for daily food iron intake for normal men and nonmenstruating women is 5 mg to 10 mg a day; for menstruating women it is 7 mg to 20 mg a day; for a pregnant woman, 20 mg to 48 mg a day; for adolescents 10 mg to 20 mg a day; for children, 4 mg to 10 mg a day and for infants, 1.5 mg per kg of body weight per day. Please carefully note this is food iron. It is bound up with organic material in your food. In this form it is absorbed only about one-tenth as well as iron that you might get as a pure salt in a pill. Therefore, with pure iron salts you require only about one-tenth these amounts.

Once again, I would like to emphasize there is evidence that the iron intake of the American, menstruating woman may be borderline. However, since it is both expensive to be on an iron supplement diet and the iron supplement might be hiding the presence of another disease, you should first be checked with a simple test, done very quickly, to determine that, indeed, you do have an iron deficiency anemia before starting to take iron supplementation.

Iron tablets are available in many forms, but the most common are ferrous sulfate, also called iron sulfate (Feosol). Other forms are ferrous fumarate, ferrous gluconate, ferrous lactate, ferrous carbonate, and ferrous chloride. The dosages are from 125 mg to 300 mg per tablet. Generally, the tablets are coated because they cause a bit of upset in the gastrointestinal system. For the best absorption, iron should not be taken in conjunction with foods. On the other hand, to prevent the gastrointestinal upset it is quite common to take the iron with other foods. You must balance between getting an adequate absorption and not getting an upset stomach from the iron salts. Since iron is a very cheap compound when bought as an individual tablet, as opposed to some of the expensive vitamin or iron supplemented mixtures, usually an excess is taken when something is eaten to stop the stomach upset. The excess amount takes care of the poor absorption factor.

Most people don't realize, when they casually begin taking iron as a food supplement, with vitamins, or when they self-diagnose an iron deficiency anemia, that iron is a toxic chemical. Luckily for the adult, it takes a rather large amount of iron to poison. To have an acute lethal effect, the dose of iron in the adult is probably about 50 gms of absorbed iron. If you will look at a bottle of iron sulfate tablets you will see that there is enough in there to kill you. On the other hand, with children, serious, acute poisoning with iron is very common. Children can die after an ingestion of as little as 1 gm of iron. This is particularly a problem since many of the colored sugar coatings on commercial iron tablets make them look like candy. This is something that people don't realize. Your bottle of vitamins, with its iron supplement, can be a lethal weapon for an infant. In the United States today there is an average of at least one death per month from the ingestion of iron by infants.

The symptoms of acute iron poisoning usually start in thirty minutes, but they can be delayed for up to several hours. It causes severe irritation of the stomach and gut, nausea, vomiting; then shock, drowsiness, diarrhea with a green stool; collapse of the heart and blood vessel system, and finally death between six and forty-eight hours. The treatment for poisoning with iron is to induce vomiting as quickly as possible to try to get the iron back up. Then, as quickly as possible, get the child to a hospital.

A problem also occurs when there is a prolonged, chronic, over-supply of iron. The body seems to stash excess iron into all sorts of tissues where it doesn't normally do so. This excessive amount of stored iron causes a condition called hemochromatosis. In this disorder, granules of iron are found in the liver, the spleen, and the bone marrow. These areas actually become iron colored. This condition is not as dangerous as the iron poisoning of children. Yet, it is not a good condition to have.

This discussion of iron can make you think about the various ads that you hear and see. Note that most of the ads do carefully state that iron is useful only when there is an established condition of iron deficiency anemia. On the other hand, there is no information included about the quick and easy test to find out whether you really do have such an anemia. Further, the ads seem to imply that males need it as much as females, which is not true, since they don't have a regular blood loss. Also, there is even the implication that older, post-menopausal women may need it as much or more than younger women. This is, of course, untrue. Finally, I don't think I've ever heard any ads point out the danger of iron poisoning, either the acute kind that happens with little children or the long-term kind in which the various tissues develop too much stored iron.

▶▶▶ VITAMIN B$_{12}$ (CYANOCOBALAMIN)

Recently vitamin B$_{12}$ has come into importance. It is closely related to iron in that it is a treatment for cases of pernicious anemia that have resulted from a lack of adequate vitamin B$_{12}$. Please note that there is a great deal of difference between pernicious anemia and iron deficiency anemia — they are two totally different conditions. Vitamin B_{12} is found in many kinds of seafoods, meat, cheeses, and so on. It is found in the greatest amount in fresh beef liver. As little as 1 gm of fresh beef liver will contain 1 mcg of vitamin B_{12}. Since the human adult requirement for B_{12} is only about 0.1 mcg per day, one-tenth of 1 gm of fresh beef liver would easily provide all that you would need. Also, fishes, meats, and cheeses contain enough to easily fulfill the requirements for B_{12}.

B_{12} is essential for normal growth and nutrition. It is involved in processes all over the body. A deficiency of B_{12} is first seen in the production of misformed red blood cells. Its lack causes an anemia. The earliest signs of a deficiency of B_{12} are numbness, tingling in the hands and feet, various neurological symptoms with poor muscular coordination, moodiness, mental slowness, poor memory, confusion, and visual problems. True pernicious anemia is a relatively rare event. It is almost impossible for the average person not to get enough B_{12} in his everyday diet. Further, many times pernicious anemia is not caused by the lack of adequate B_{12} intake, but rather, the lack of other chemicals that are needed to work with B_{12} so it can function correctly in the body. The only reason for taking B_{12} in amounts in excess of the normal dietary intake is to cure pernicious anemia due to a specifically diagnosed B_{12} deficiency. It has no good effects on its own. It is a very highly specialized vitamin although a very important one for the body. Fortunately, since pure B_{12} is being sold across the counter, it does not have toxic reactions when taken orally, and even when injected, it will rarely cause even an allergic reaction.

▶▶ FOLIC ACID (PTEROYLGLUTAMIC ACID)

A chemical similar to B_{12} that is also involved in the production of red blood cells is folic acid (pteroylglutamic acid). This chemical is found in many common foods. There is no reason for it to be taken, except in cases of specific proven deficiency of folic acid. It is also easily obtainable across the counter. The recommended intake is 50 mcg daily for adults, 15 mcg for infants, 100 mcg for children, and 400 mcg during pregnancy. It can be obtained as folic acid (Folvite) or folinic acid (Citrovorum factor Leucovorin). Its only known use is for an established deficiency of folic acid that is related to pernicious anemia. Generally, it is easy to get an adequate quantity in the diet. Liver and spinach have a particularly high content of this chemical. Folic acid is also nontoxic in man, so you cannot harm yourself by taking too much of it. On the other hand, its presence in the multivitamin mixtures and as tablets probably involves a waste of money.

A subject that should be mentioned briefly is the so-called "megavitamin" therapy. This is a theory that is espoused by certain organic food believers and a few very prominent scientists, such as Linus Pauling. They have proposed that large doses, perhaps thousands or millions times the usual dose, of the nontoxic, water-soluble vitamins might help prevent colds, cure mental disease, aid athletic performance, and provide a myriad of other benefits. The evidence to support these claims is very sparse and very controversial. However, there is always the chance that they may be right. Only time and a lot more scientific data will prove or disprove the claims. For now, I think I'll stick to the more conservative view that only vitamin deficiencies require vitamin supplementation. The data on the use of vitamin C in high doses to reduce the symptoms of a cold may be an exception to this general statement.

To summarize the use of vitamin and mineral supplements in the diet, a few general points should be made. First, if you have an adequate diet you don't need any of them. They are a waste of your money. Fortunately, not too many of these chemicals are harmful even in vast excess of the required amounts. The only time you need supplementation of your diet is when it is proven that you have a deficiency, and then it is usually reasonably easy and inexpensive to bring your body pools of the vitamin back up. Second, some of the compounds are toxic if taken in extreme amounts. Particularly to be watched are vitamins A and D, and iron. Calcium too can be dangerous but not as often. Finally, consider the information that has been discussed here, then listen to and read the ads that are produced by the mass media. It's not truly "false" advertising but it surely is tricky and misleading. Let the buyer beware.

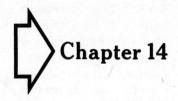

Chapter 14

Drugs for the Skin

Each year the American public spends between two and five million dollars for various ointments, creams, lotions, medications, powders, and sprays to apply to the skin. The purpose of this massive spreading of chemicals on the skin varies from a desire to have soft, "silky" skin, to cure acne and dandruff, or to remove corns and warts. Most people don't think of these chemicals as drugs. Rather, they use the term "moisturizing cream," or "wrinkle remover," or some other expression to describe these chemicals. But the fact of the matter is they are active chemicals and are placed on the body with the expectation of some beneficial biological result. Therefore, they are drugs.

The particular compound that a specific manufacturer produces is generally a mixture of a number of different types of chemicals, each of which, they hope, will confer a specific benefit upon the user, the combination being the optimal mixture to provide the desired overall result. The rationale for some of these mixtures is sometimes very difficult to understand and, indeed, quite often all of the individual components could be easily replaced by other chemicals with no particular change in action. Each manufacturer treasures his own particular mixture and I'm sure each thinks his own is the best. But, when considering these mixtures from the point of view of pharmacology, for the most part, they vary more in perfume, color, and price than in any important way of working. It would be next to impossible to choose one particular mixture over another on the basis of the chemicals it contains.

▶▶▶ THE NATURE OF THE SKIN

In order to understand the way drugs work upon the skin, you must understand something about the skin itself. Skin is a very useful type of tissue. It is a protective sheath that serves to keep your bodily fluids in and to keep germs out.

The outermost layer of the skin is composed of a dead sheath of cells that were once living. These serve as a protective coat for your body. This outside husk, or sheath, of cells is composed mainly of a protein called keratin. As the cells on the inner surface are pushed outward by new cells, the older ones die. They then deposit their outside husk, composed of keratin, to form a hard, crusty, protective layer for your skin. This is a constant process. In daily living, you are constantly scratching, rubbing, or abrading the outside layer of dead keratin. This layer is being continually replaced, as the inner, living cells of the skin die and are pushed outward to the surface. Also, moisture is steadily drawn up from the living cells deeper in the skin to give at least a 10 percent water content to the hard, keratin layer. It is the moisture content of the keratin layer that makes the skin feel soft.

In the skin are follicles from which hair grows. Hair is composed of the protein keratin, just as the outside layer of skin is. However, in hair, the keratin is stretched into a long, complex organization of the protein. In association with the hair follicles are three types of glands. One, which opens directly into the top of the hair follicle, is called sebaceous. The function of the sebaceous glands is to produce a fatty substance called sebum. The sebum produced by the sebaceous glands goes out through the top of the hair follicle and coats the outside of the keratin layer. The purpose of this oily, fatty sebum is first, to provide a lubricant for the skin and second, to prevent the water in the keratinous layer from being evaporated too quickly into the air. This means that if you have an inadequate amount of sebum on your skin, either from a lack of production or because you've washed it all off, the skin can become very dry and will crack and peel.

The other two types of glands associated with the skin and hair follicles are the apocrine and eccrine sweat glands. The eccrine sweat glands produce sweat predominantly in response to heat. By producing sweat, which is then evaporated, the body cools itself. The average person produces between one and three pints of sweat each day, even though he is generally not aware that he is perspiring. This is a necessary mechanism for the body. Without the ability to sweat you would quickly go into a severe fever and die from overheating. The apocrine sweat glands are a bit different. They are separate glands. They produce a different kind of sweat. The apocrine sweat glands produce sweat when you are under stress or emotional strain. They are not very responsive to heat. This is the kind of sweat that, when broken down chemically by various types of germs that normally reside on the skin, produces the unpleasant odor that most of us try to eliminate or cover with deodorants and antiperspirants. The apocrine glands produce sweat constantly even though you are not under tension but their greatest action is during situations of emotional stress.

People are endowed with varying amounts of hair, produce varying amounts of sebum, and have differing numbers of the two types of sweat glands. This is why some people seem to have problems with dandruff, called "seborrhea capitis." This term means "problems with the sebaceous glands in the head." Acne is another condition related to the sebaceous glands. People differ in regard to this disorder also. Some have it much worse than others. Fortunately, we all change with time. Acne in the fourteen-to-twenty-year age bracket is almost universal. But, for most people the acne eventually goes away all by itself.

▶▶ PROBLEMS OF THE SKIN

Various unpleasant problems are associated with the skin and, unfortunately, very little is known about any of them. One is acne. In this condition apparently there is a change in the chemical nature of the sebum so that instead of being composed mostly of very large fat molecules, smaller fat molecules are present. The large fat molecules of the sebum are broken down into other, smaller fats, due to the action of your body, and possibly, the action of germs. The presence of these small fat molecules can cause the sebaceous glands to react as though they were being invaded by infecting germs. There really isn't any such invasion, but the body reacts as if there were. The sebaceous glands then become inflamed. The bodily defenses against infection rush to the site and, in general, act just as if there had been a bacterial invasion. It is this inflammation that we call acne. It is a false alarm to the body's infection fighting brigade. Sometimes, particular germs can be present also. These non-oxygen-using germs can also contribute to acne.

Another common disorder of the skin is associated with the presence of either too little or too much sebum, causing either dry skin or overly oily skin. Your hands or your face may get chapped and raw, or conversely, you may feel greasy all the time. If this happens to your scalp, the odds are that you will have dandruff. Dandruff seems to be associated with either the under- or over-production of sebum. However, very little is known about dandruff, and there is probably a good deal more to the problem than just sebum production.

Two other disorders quite closely related to dandruff are called "eczema" and "psoriasis." These are general terms that describe a condition of chapping, reddening, roughing, and flaking of skin tissue. We have no idea what causes this kind of condition. All we can hope for is some form of symptomatic treatment: not a cure but possibly some relief.*

Also, there are corns, which can be called "ingrown calluses." Corns are caused in the same manner as the calluses you get on your hands when you work. They come from mechanical pressure due to badly fitting shoes, or some other source of friction and pressure. In both corns and calluses there is a growth of the keratin layer into a hard lump that can penetrate deep into the inner levels of the skin. The keratin growth begins to push on nerve endings deep in the skin. This hurts. The corn is composed of the same material as the outer keratin layer of the skin, except that it is in a big lump and invades deeper levels of the skin.

Warts are caused by viruses. There are probably a number of types of viruses that can cause warts, some of which are communicable by touch. It is not wise to go around rubbing other people's warts. The wart is tissue very much like tissue of a corn except it is raised and is due to a viral infection, not pressure.

The final skin condition I will discuss is a cosmetic one. Many people seem to wish to have soft, "silky" skin, whatever that means. And, most people object to having harsh, chapped skin. Indeed, dryness and cracking do open up the skin and break down the protective layer that skin forms against invading germs. Prickly rashes, due to sweat, and diaper rashes, due to the absence of an adequate amount of sebum, are similar cases of the breakdown of the protective layer of the skin. In diaper rash, the ammonia from the baby's urine causes a washing away of the sebum. Then the mechanical irritation of the diaper abrades the skin, which causes a rash to form.

---

* Ultraviolet light treatment of these conditions is showing some progress toward a true "cure."

Drugs that are used for the skin are categorized in terms of their functions in relation to the skin. However, most commercial preparations will be mixtures of two or more of these drugs with the hope of attaining the ideal combination for the particular result desired. Further, each of these chemicals tends to have more than one kind of action on the skin so that to classify them under only one heading is an over-simplification. However, in discussing these drugs we will talk about them in terms of their major actions only.

Demulcents

Demulcents are a group of chemicals used to coat the skin to reduce irritation. They are particularly good on tender surfaces such as mucous membrane in the nose or throat, but they can also be used to protect skin areas that have been scraped open or have been mechanically harmed. They are in lozenges and gargles for sore throats since they can coat the throat and help reduce the irritation. They are also found in lotions, ointments, and dressings for scrapes and scars, and they are used to mask the taste of a drug, as perfume masks the odor of a drug.

Perhaps the oldest known demulcent is acacia (gum arabic). This can be used as a powder or a syrup. It is generally incorporated into lozenges and gargles. Tragacanth (gum tragacanth) has similar properties and uses. Other chemicals in this group from natural sources are: glycyrrhiza (licorice root), agar, sodium alginate, methylcellulose, and sodium carboxymethyl cellulose. Synthetic chemicals used to coat and protect the skin are glycerols such as glycerin, propylene glycol, polyethylene glycol, and diethylene glycol. It should be noted that the glycerins and glycols can only be used on the outside of the skin, not on mucous tissues, since they are absorbed and are poisonous. Finally, a new drug that is classed as a demulcent but also has other properties is allantoin. This is a synthetically produced chemical that was originally discovered in a number of natural products. Synethetic production reduces the cost.

Emollients

Emollients are lubricants. They act by substituting for sebum that has been washed away. Therefore, like sebum, they are fats or oils. Emollients are components found in all moisturizing creams, cold creams, and similar cosmetics and lotions. They provide lubrication of the skin and, by replacing the sebum, aid the keratin layer of the skin in retaining its moisture and, thereby, a soft and flexible character. The usual emollients are cottonseed oil, olive oil, almond oil, corn oil, persic oil, peanut oil, theobroma oil (cocoa butter), lanolin, mineral oil, paraffin, petroleum, petroleum jelly, beeswax, spermaceti, and various combinations of these. For example, a common emollient is rose water ointment. It consists of spermaceti, white wax, almond oil, rose water, and rose oil. This is the usual sort of base you will find in any "cold cream."

Another group of emollient compounds are bath oils. These are particularly useful if the fatty oil emollients are combined with a detergent. This mixture will cause the bath oil to be dispersed on the top of your bath water. This means that when you get out of the bathtub you will pick up a thin film of the oil, which, if you do not towel too vigorously, will serve as an excellent protective layer to replace the sebum that you have just washed off. Antichapping and antisunburn pomades, lotions, and creams are also mostly mixtures of various emollients. True, ultraviolet-light-filtering "sunscreens" also contain para-aminobenzoic acid or its derivatives. The presence of this chemical helps prevent burning but still allows tanning by a filtration of most ultraviolet radiation.

Protectives

Protectives are generally powders that serve to reduce irritation from a mechanical source. For example, the dusting powder that you use on a baby's bottom to reduce the friction caused by a diaper is a protective. It has the same sort of function as spreading powdered graphite on the moving parts of a machine. Further, some of these protective powders have other properties such as being mildly antiseptic. This can be helpful if there is a problem with the invasion by germs of the abraded area. However, these powders tend to crust and can inhibit wound healing. You should be cautioned, however, that these kinds of powders can be absorbed into the blood if there is an open wound, a burned spot, a rash, or an abraded area. When absorbed into the body a number of these powders are toxic substances. Therefore, you should be careful to use dusting powders only on intact skin. They are best used to prevent mechanical abrasion, not to cure it.

The common protective dusting powders are zinc oxide, ferrous oxide, a combination of half zinc oxide and half ferrous oxide (calamine), zinc stearate, magnesium stearate, starch, boric acid, and talc (which is predominantly magnesium silicate). Cooked oatmeal is also a good, cheap protective. It is sponged onto the body from a cloth bag.

Astringents and Antiperspirants

Astringents and antiperspirants are chemicals that cause the skin at the top of the hair follicles and the sweat glands to become slightly enlarged and very mildly inflamed. This tends to stop the secretion of sweat and sebum and to cause a tightening of the skin as a whole. The same property of the drug that tightens the skin on your face when used in an astringent stops perspiration under the arms when used in an antiperspirant. It seals off the sweat glands, which reduces the wetness and, particularly with the apocrine sweat glands, odor. All of these chemicals can cause allergic reactions in some people.

The common astringents presently used are alum, aluminum subacetate, aluminum acetate, aluminum chloride, aluminum chlorhydrate, aluminum sulfate, aluminum formate, aluminum hydroxychloride, aluminum hydroxide, zinc oxide, aluminum sulfocarbolate, and zinc phenolsulfonate. Further, aluminum chlorhydroxide can be formed into a complex chemical called chlorhydrol. Aluminum chlorhydroxy lactate (chloracel) is sometimes used in antiperspirant sticks. Glutaraldehyde is a new, very potent antiperspirant.

Formerly, various types of natural products that contained tannic acid were used as astringents. These came from the nuts of the oak, rose, witch hazel, sumac, chestnut, and other plants. However, the tannins are no longer used in most products, since they have been found to be poisonous to the liver if absorbed. Tannins were also used for burns, for example, soaking the burned area with wet tea leaves, but due to their poisonous properties, this practice is now discouraged.

The astringents have a second property in addition to causing a mild swelling at the surface of the various openings for hair, sweat, and sebaceous glands. They can cause a living skin cell to die. However, they have a very low penetration rate through the skin and, therefore, can only affect the cells that are quite close to the surface — those right under the horny keratin layer. This action leads to a hardening of the skin by causing a more rapid production of dead material for the keratin layer. At the same time, they will cause a hardening of the surfaces of the small blood vessels close to the surface of the skin. This is particularly effective if you put an astringent directly onto mucous tissue. This hardening of the capillary surface can help stop mild bleeding. Thus, astringents used as styptic pencils can help relieve some of the discomfort of inflamed or abraded mucous membranes, such as are present in hemorrhoids.

Deodorants

Deodorants are of two types. First, there are the various perfumes that we use to mask our body odors. These will not be discussed since they have no true pharmacological effect but are used only to please. The second class of deodorants is antiseptics. These compounds, which we have previously discussed, act to kill the germs on the skin that are responsible for the breakdown of the products in apocrine sweat that give it its unpleasant odor. The common deodorant antiseptics are benzalkonium fluoride, hexachlorophene, tyrothricin, neomycin, and methylbenzethonium chloride. Each of these has its own particular disadvantages and advantages. Methonium type derivatives, for example, benzalkonium or methylbenzethonium, are inactivated by soap and will irritate the skin if used in greater than a 1 percent concentration. The use of an antibiotic, like neomycin, can result in either the production of resistant strains of germs, or, in some people, allergic reactions. Hexachlorophene can penetrate through the skin to yield blood levels that are worrisome in terms of causing poisoning. The advantage of each deodorant is the degree to which it kills germs and the length of time it acts. These properties were discussed in the chapter on antiseptics.

Keratolytics

Keratolytic compounds cause a sloughing of the keratin layer of the skin. This exposes the lower, live levels of cells to the outside. This breakdown of the protective keratin coat then causes the live cells to die, which produces a new keratin layer. As the cells exposed to the outside die, new cells are formed. It's rather like shedding your old skin to get a new one. This process can be quite useful when trying to get the penetration of an antifungal drug or an antiseptic into the real source of an infection deep under the keratin layer. It is also of aid in causing the drying up of excessive oiliness and will help eliminate flakiness of some skin disorders. These "flakes" are only large, organized bits of keratin. The keratolytics are all relatively potent and poisonous chemicals, however. Most of them are absorbable through the skin. Therefore, their use must be confined to relatively small areas and used only on intact, unburned skin. Otherwise, you might get poisoned from them.

The standard keratolytic agents are salicylic acid, salicylamide, benzoic acid, resorcinol, sulfur, phenol, and camphor. On the whole, the use of the keratolytic agents to soften and loosen skin and to cause the keratin layer to slough off can probably be thought of as scraping yourself all over with a dull knife. The ancient Greeks took baths this way. They oiled themselves and then were scraped with dull knives. This is essentially what the keratolytic agents do. Of course, the Greeks, after being scraped down, re-oiled themselves with an emollient, as should be done after using a keratolytic drug.

A very specific keratolytic agent that is used for the treatment of dandruff is selenium sulfide (Selsun). Selenium sulfide is a highly toxic substance when orally ingested. Further, prolonged contact with the skin can cause severe burns. However, not much of it is absorbed through the skin. When it is used in a therapeutic shampoo there is about 2.5 percent selenium sulfide in combination with a detergent. You wash your hair with it, leave it on five to ten minutes, and then very carefully rinse it off. Be sure to keep it away from your eyes since it can be very irritating. This procedure will be successful in most cases if performed once or twice a week. About 95 percent of the cases of simple dandruff are controlled by the treatment. Selenium sulfide acts by causing a sloughing off of the flaky keratin layer of the scalp. This exposes fresh skin to the outside.

The procedure has some objectionable features. It is a little difficult to do — you have to be very careful that you don't get selenium sulfide in your eyes or ears. You must not keep it on the skin too long and be sure not to swallow any. Finally, it may turn gray hair somewhat orange and sometimes can cause excessive hair loss and an over-oiliness of the scalp. A similar type of chemical used as a dandruff treatment is cadmium sulfide (Capsebon). It is used in just about the same way as selenium sulfide. Sulfur compounds are also used as antidandruff agents. They act in the same way.

Detergents

Detergents are synthetic, acidic chemicals that act in the same general way that soap does, that is, they help water get close enough to oil and dirt to rinse them away. However, soap is alkaline and forms insoluble salts in hard water that can coat the hair and dull its gloss. It can also coat the skin. The synthetic detergents are almost all based on the chemical laurylic acid. You'll see this in many forms. It could be lauryl isoquinoline bromide, sodium lauryl sulfate, triethanolamine lauryl sulfate, or many other similar forms. However, they all act in about the same way. They, like soap, get water right down to the spot where it can wash. To do this, they cut through oily and fatty substances. From this action you can see that detergents, or soaps for that matter, will have both good and bad properties. First, they will cut fats and oils. This is why they help wash your dishes. On the other hand, they will also remove the sebum from your skin since it too is a fat. Thus, they can cause harshness and drying. The keratin layer is no longer protected by sebum so its moisture will be evaporated. On the other hand, detergents and soaps clean to allow other drugs to get to where they need to go, under the keratin layer, to get the effect that you want. It is for these reasons that many of the modern detergents are balanced by combining emollients with them. Thus, while you are washing off your own sebum, you are replacing it with a substitute fat emollient.

In a shampoo there will usually be other ingredients, such as a foaming agent, as well as a detergent. Foaming agents help clean an area by causing bubbles to be formed. The bubbles mechanically lift the particles out to help clean. Finally, many products are a combination of different kinds of detergents. Sometimes the manufacturer will even balance acidic detergents with organic alkaline materials so that the alkaline-acidity balance can be kept just about neutral. Precisely how important that is to its action is impossible to say but it certainly helps the sales campaigns. Adding protein to hair products falls into the same category: probably more advertising value than pharmacological value.

To summarize, cleaning aids will probably be a combination of a detergent or a soap or both to get good cleaning action, with an emollient to protect the keratin layer and keep it soft. Quite often they will contain an antiseptic to reduce the active number of germs on the body to help to deodorize.

Caustics and Depilatories

Caustics are used only for the removal of warts and corns. Caustics are actually very strong keratolytic agents, for they remove the protein. As they get around the edges of your corn or wart, they will cause it to soften and, eventually, to fall or be pushed out as the tissue is sloughed away and new cells are produced. Because of this strong keratolytic action, you have to be very careful to confine the action of the caustic to just the area of the wart or the corn. The usual caustics are trichloroacetic acid, glacial acetic acid, lactic acid, zinc chloride, silver nitrate, and salicylic acid.

Depilatories are another type of caustic preparation used on the skin. They act by causing a breakdown in one particular type of chemical of which keratin is composed. Keratin has approximately 17 percent cystine in it. A depilatory causes a breakdown in cystine. Since the base of the hair is its least hardened part, a chemical that produces a breakdown of cystine will cause the hair to break away close to the opening of the follicle. However, if you kept a depilatory chemical on the hair long enough, the entire hair would break down and dissolve. You should remember that the outer layer of skin, as well as the hair, is made up of keratin. This should be a warning. At the same time that you remove the hair, you are going to be removing a good part of the outside layer of your skin. A depilatory is an extremely strong keratolytic agent. Further, the fatty substance, sebum, that covers the skin also covers the hair.

Before a depilatory can be truly effective the sebum must be removed. Thus, most depilatory compounds contain a detergent to remove the sebum as well as either calcium thioglycolate, barium sulfide, or calcium hydroxide as the strong keratolytic agents to provide the depilatory action. Also, great care must be taken not to exceed the time limit for the depilatory to stay on the skin. If kept on too long, you can cause permanent damage. Finally, it is wise to coat the skin with an emollient, after using a depilatory to remove hair, in order to protect the skin by replacing the sebum with an artificial lubricant. Again, as a final caution, some people do have allergic reactions to the chemicals used in depilatories. Therefore, you must be careful not to get a bad rash while removing hair.

Tetracycline

An interesting, rather different skin drug that is sometimes used in the treatment of severe acne is tetracycline. This involves a daily dose of 250 mg of the antibiotic. However, this dose level is too low for the drug to act on germs. It is believed that even very low doses of tetracycline can prevent the formation in the sebaceous glands of the particular types of fatty acids that are responsible for the inflammation of acne. This treatment method is not effective in all cases but can result in a very dramatic improvement in certain people.

Two types of problems can be associated with tetracycline therapy for acne. First, allergic reactions can be developed as I have already discussed. Second, taking such a low dose of tetracycline for long periods of time will probably result in the development of resistant germs in your body. Then, if a severe, life threatening infection develops, you probably won't be able to use tetracycline. However, there are other antibiotics that could be used in such a case. So, all in all, for people who have severe acne, this unexpected additional use of tetracycline is a real benefit. This situation also illustrates that drugs do a number of very different kinds of things in your body all at the same time. We should never forget that drugs do not only what was specifically intended but a lot of other things, too — some of which you may not like. No drug is an unmixed evil or an unmixed blessing.

Clindamycin

A more recent drug for use in acne is the antibiotic clindamycin (Cleocin) at a dose of 150 mg to 600 mg a day. This drug has a specific effect on germs that do not need oxygen to live. One theory of acne holds that these kinds of germs are responsible for the breakdown of sebum into the wrong kinds of fats that result in an allergic reaction. Whether or not this is the reason for acne, the drug does seem to work in some cases. Of course, as with any antibiotic, drug allergy has to be considered.

Combination Skin Remedies

Anti-Acne Preparations

Now that we have discussed the properties of the chemicals used individually on the skin, let's consider what might be found in some common medications. For example, an anti-acne preparation. A usual anti-acne preparation will have something to get rid of sebum since it is the breakdown of sebum that causes the problem. It will also probably have at least one, and possibly more, mild keratolytic agents, to allow the medication to get to the inflamed area. As much of the protein as possible has to be eliminated from the inflamed area so the chemicals can get into it. It will probably have an antiseptic of some kind to reduce the chances of infection and also to try to kill germs that might have aided in the breakdown of the sebum. Commonly, it will have a counterirritant type of external analgesic to help increase blood flow to the area. Finally, it will probably have a demulcent or protective powder to coat and protect the area. In addition, there may be a coloring product to hide the inflammation while, hopefully, it is going away. Therefore, a reasonably common type of anti-acne cream might contain .08 percent sulfur, 2 percent resorcinol, 2 percent salicylic acid, 1 percent hexachlorophene, as the keratolytic and antiseptic agents. It could have lauryl ether as a detergent, some menthol and camphor as mild irritants, and zinc sulfate as a protective. Finally, the whole preparation may be carried in an alcohol vehicle.

Cream for Eczema or Psoriasis

We might find in a standard cream for eczema or psoriasis a combination of a detergent to wash the area, a keratolytic to help get rid of keratin flakes, an emollient to protect the area, smooth it out, or at least make it feel smooth, possibly a counterirritant as an anti-itch compound, and finally an antiseptic added for good measure. For instance a compound for use as a cream for eczema might contain as an anti-itch one of the tars such as coal, pine, or juniper tar, or benzocaine or phenol; hexachlorophene as an antiseptic; benzoic acid as a keratolytic agent to get rid of the scales; and lanolin, as an emollient. In most ways, this differs very little from an anti-acne cream.

Dandruff Cream

A dandruff cream might contain first a keratolytic agent, perhaps 2 percent salicylic acid, or 3 percent sulfur; a mild irritant and itch reducer such as coal tar, at 2.5 percent; hexachlorophene at 1 percent as an antiseptic; lauryl ether as a detergent to get the area clean; and finally, lanolin as an emollient to recoat the surface. Again this is not much different from anti-acne creams or the "cures" for psoriasis and eczema.

Moisturizer

A "moisturizer," or "dry skin cosmetic," will contain a perfume, some type of emollient because this will fill in the little troughs in the skin thus making it feel softer, and possibly some vitamin A. If it is a medicated cream it will contain an antiseptic. The use of vitamins A or D is relatively new in this field. Some studies have indicated that there may be some benefit from vitamins A or D, either for acne or, generally, in helping the skin heal itself. However, the evidence is very sparse at present that these vitamins help in any way at all.

Mixture for Diaper Rash

For a mixture for diaper rash, we might find an antiseptic, such as hexachlorophene, again, perhaps, with vitamin A or vitamin D, just in case it might help. The diaper rash powder might contain zinc oxide as a protective; again, not too different from any of the other skin chemicals we have discussed.

In general, whenever you are dealing with the skin, first wash it with a detergent or soap to strip off the sebum. Then, in order to penetrate with other chemicals and remove flakes or the old horny layer, use a keratolytic agent. Next, an astringent, to cause a tightening of the skin and a fresh keratin layer to be exposed. With a fresh layer of skin exposed, coat the skin with an artificial sebum in the form of an emollient, and finally a powder to give a protective coating to the skin to reduce its sensitivity to friction. The precise amounts and percentages of different chemicals, keratolytics, astringents, or emollients depend upon which of the particular conditions you are trying to treat.

Fundamentally, almost all of the compounds used on the skin have the same chemicals and, to a large extent, the same properties. From a pharmacological viewpoint one particular combination is probably about as effective as another. The greatest single factor in your choice will probably be your own aesthetic taste, the cost, the feel, the odor, or some other property of the particular chemical combination that you choose.

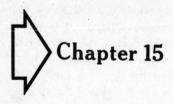

Chapter 15

Drugs and the Kidney (Diuretics)

Diuretics are taken when there is a need to have the body put out more water in the urine and when the amount of water in body tissue should be decreased. There are a number of illnesses in which water can accumulate in the body to an excessive extent. Heart failure causes edema, that is, swelling of the ankles and other parts of the body, and sometimes even puffiness of the legs. Sometimes cirrhosis of the liver causes watery fluid to collect in the abdomen. This excess water is undesirable and has to be removed. In the case of water in the abdomen after cirrhosis, a physician might make an opening in the stomach wall to let the fluid out directly. However, it is much better to have the kidneys put out the fluid instead. Kidney failure is another serious condition in which water backs up in the body. Drugs do not help kidney failure.

A cautionary note: anyone who has major swelling of the belly or the lower extremities, or has diffuse puffiness of unknown cause throughout the body should see his doctor and shouldn't borrow a diuretic from a friend. Diuretic medication taken on top of failing kidneys can make a person much sicker.

There are two conditions in which diuretics are widely used by some doctors and widely scorned by others. These are dieting for weight loss and premenstrual tension, both in women who are not taking contraceptive pills and women who are and may be storing additional water in their tissues.

▶▶▶ PROBLEMS OF OVERWEIGHT

In the case of weight loss, there is no evidence that taking a diuretic drug actually makes anybody lose any *permanent* weight. The diuretic causes the loss of water, not fat. However, taking a diuretic will often make a person lose 2 to 4 pounds at the beginning of the diet. This can give the person a psychological feeling that the diet is successful. The person, of course, must continue taking the diuretic pills for a prolonged period or he will gain back the 2 to 4 pounds in water weight as soon as he stops. Whether or not this illusory extra loss of weight is worthwhile to encourage people to stick to a strict diet is a matter of conjecture. Some people who have gone on prolonged diets swear that taking diuretics helps them in the long haul as well as over the first few days. I know of no evidence to support this claim but, again, doctor's opinions vary. One note of caution should be introduced, however. There are some doctors who specialize in weight reduction who use a wide variety of drugs to make people lose weight very rapidly. Although a low dose of a diuretic may be all right, there is a point at which combinations of diuretics, plus thyroid hormones, amphetamines, digitalis, and so on, can, in fact, produce serious harm. One might well be wary when going to a doctor who distributes his own pills, that is, does not prescribe through drugstores, or one who is reluctant to give detailed information as to exactly what he is prescribing and why.

▶▶▶ PREMENSTRUAL TENSION

In the case of premenstrual tension, many women seek relief from the painful or uncomfortable swelling of the breasts and, often, the abdomen, ankles, and other parts of the body, that often occurs just before a menstrual period and may persist throughout. Although hormone and other treatments have been tried for premenstrual tension, many women feel that diuretic drugs not only decrease their physical discomfort but also may decrease the severity of cramps that they may have during a period. Again, doctors have differing views about prescribing diuretic drugs to relieve this relatively common source of discomfort for women.

It seems to me that the decrease in discomfort with a relatively safe drug is well worth the relatively small risk attached at least to the benzothiadiazide diuretics. Doctors will place varying emphasis on benefits gained versus risks encountered. Some diuretics will change the amount of sodium and potassium in the blood in an undesirable manner. Also, occasionally, people can have allergic reactions to these drugs, as they can to almost any other drug. In addition, if there is a tendency toward gout, drugs of this sort could increase the amount of uric acid in the blood. This might produce an attack of gout, though it seems a bit unlikely. Similarly, if a borderline diabetic takes these drugs, they will slightly increase the amount of glucose in the blood. This action may push you over into clinically apparent diabetes. The odds of any of these things happening seem to be small enough to make the comfort worth the risk. However, if one is to use these drugs at all regularly, it is necessary to have a thorough physical examination first. Also, find a doctor who feels comfortable prescribing these drugs in a careful and watchful manner. Again, you and your doctor must get together to evaluate whether the amount of discomfort you get with your menstrual period is worth the modest risk attached to the use of oral diuretic drugs. It is not worth taking any drug for relatively minor discomfort, but if you really are quite uncomfortable and your dress size changes substantially just before your period, it seems to me that the use of a diuretic may be considered if you have no physical condition that makes it contraindicated.

▶▶▶ ACTIONS OF DIURETIC DRUGS

First, there are two meanings of the word "diuretic." It can mean a substance used to increase the amount of urine. This can be water, beer, coffee, or almost any fluid in large amounts. With the exception of coffee, these fluids do not, in fact, change the amount of fluid that you are holding in and around your body cells and in your blood. They just cause you to pass a lot more water while you remain essentially unchanged by all this fluid passage. Of course, if you drink a really huge amount of water you can, in fact, die of water poisoning, but, except for this extreme case, you are very unlikely to get in any particular trouble or change yourself much. This kind of fast flushing with water can be helpful when you are taking sulfa drugs or for some kidney infections.

Caffeine in coffee acts in a somewhat different way. It decreases the reabsorption of sodium and chloride into the blood from the tubes in the kidneys. Therefore, it is a real diuretic, though less potent than the benzothiadiazide drugs.

The more usual sense of the word "diuretic," as it has been used in this chapter so far, is a drug that will pull both water and various salts, chiefly sodium chloride, out of your body in significant amounts so that the amount of water in the tissues is decreased. Your tissues, in fact, get drier. Any extra water that may have accumulated in your ankles, feet, or abdomen is pulled out and leaves your body via the urine. This involves the mechanics of osmotic pressure. Any two fluids separated by a membrane that will only let through very small molecules, like water, will adjust themselves so that the amount of pressure on each side of the membrane is equal. Maintaining the pressure on each side of the membrane is a function of the chemicals dissolved in the fluid. For example, if you put a very concentrated solution of sugar on one side of a membrane and a very weak solution of sugar on the other side, the osmotic pressure of the concentrated sugar solution will pull water out of the weak sugar solution until the solutions on both sides of the membrane have the same sugar concentration. Their osmotic pressures are then equal. In your body, this osmotic pressure, in part, is caused by the protein material in your blood, in the fluids around your cells, and inside your cells. Also, a large part of the osmotic pressure in your body is contributed by the electrolytes. "Electrolytes" is the term for salt ions that are dissolved in body fluids. The common ones and highest in concentration are sodium, chloride, potassium, and hydrogen. The relative concentrations of these ions in your cells, in the area surrounding your cells, and in your blood determine how water will be distributed in your body.

The kidneys are made up of a large number of individual filtering systems called nephrons. At one end of each nephron is an area where the pressure of the blood pushes fluid out of the blood into the kidney tubes. These kidney tubes go through a number of swirls and squiggles where sodium and chloride are absorbed out of or pumped back into the blood until just the right amounts of these ions are retained in the body. The walls of the tubes act like inert membranes allowing higher osmotic pressure on one side or the other to pull fluid in or out. The kidney tubes also have special ways of actively pumping ions one way or the other as well as using osmotic pressure to adjust fluid and ion concentration. The sum of all this activity of the kidneys is to carefully adjust the body fluid's concentration of sodium, chloride, potassium, and hydrogen ions. At the same time, the kidneys are balancing the amount of body fluid. They are also putting out waste material, such as urea left over from proteins burned as fuel, which would otherwise poison the system. As you may recall, probenecid acts to reduce gout by inhibiting the reabsorption of uric acid in the kidneys. This is an example of how some drugs work by changing the adjustment of the kidneys.

Diuresis, that is, elimination of excess water, can be obtained by putting something into your body that will change the osmotic pressure between blood and kidney tubes. Mannitol, a sugar-like substance that is not metabolized in the body, is such a substance. Mannitol is pushed out of the blood into the kidney tubes. There it stays. It can't be reabsorbed. Since it can't be reabsorbed, its osmotic pressure sucks fluid out of the body to compensate. This makes more fluid go out in the urine. This kind of diuretic is not usually used in outpatients under ordinary circumstances. These are called "osmotic" diuretics since they work strictly by osmotic pressure. They give the clearest picture of how osmotic pressure changes regulate body water level.

Benzothiadiazide Diuretics

The commonest kind of diuretics used for outpatients are the benzothiadiazides. The most widely used of these are chlorothiazide (Diuril) 500 mg to 2000 mg per day, hydrochlorothiazide (Hydrodiuril, Esidrix) 25 mg to 100 mg per day, bendroflumethiazide (Rauzide) 2 mg to 5 mg per day, benzthiazide (Exna) 25 mg to 50 mg per day, polythiazide (Renese) 4 mg to 8 mg per day, cyclothiazide (Anhydron) 1 mg to 6 mg per day, methyclothiazide (Enduron) 5 mg to 8 mg per day, and trichlormethiazide (Naqua) 4 mg to 8 mg per day. These drugs and others like them act by interfering with the reabsorption of sodium and chloride ions from the kidney tubes. Water will follow the sodium and chloride out of the blood to rebalance osmotic pressure. However, at the same time, they pump potassium out of the body. Sometimes, when they are given in too large amounts or too often, they pump out more potassium than is good for your body to lose. Under those circumstances your heart action can be altered a bit and you can feel wrung out, weak, and peculiar. For these reasons, some companies make diuretic pills that include potassium salts to replenish your supply. These are now frowned upon by many physicians since the pills tend to dissolve in one spot in the small intestine. This causes a high concentration of potassium that can sometimes burn a small hole in the wall of the gut, causing a lot of secondary troubles. If potassium is prescribed along with a diuretic, it is usually given either in a liquid form or in some form that will be dissolved in the stomach rather than in the small intestine.

As will be noted in the section on heart drugs, benzothiadiazides also have the property of reducing high blood pressure. They may do this by affecting sodium and chloride excretion, though this is uncertain. The bezothiadiazide drugs have been prescribed for high blood pressure patients who take them every day, for long periods of time, even years, without encountering serious side effects. This apparent safety is one of the reasons I feel relatively comfortable in having such drugs prescribed to relieve such conditions as premenstrual tension or to initiate weight loss in patients who are otherwise physically healthy. Check with your own doctor, however, before embarking on anything like this.

There are several other types of diuretic chemicals. Most of them are very strong and not used too often. A few are: mercury diuretics, such as calomel, merbaphen (Novasurol), and mersalyl (Salyrgan); nonmercury diuretics, such as acetazolamide (Diamox), ethacrynic acid (Edecrin), furosemide (Lasix), and spironolactone (Aldactone). Triamterene (Dyrenium) is a drug that is mildly diuretic but helps the body retain potassium. It is often used in combination with hydrochlorothiazide so that no potassium supplement is required. This combination is called Dyazide. With Dyazide one must watch for an excess of potassium in the blood.

Chapter 16

Drugs and the Heart

In order to understand how drugs affect the heart it is first necessary to understand something about the heart itself. The heart is a
large, muscular pump that pushes blood through the body. In fact,
it is two pumps; one side of the heart pumps blood through the
lungs, where the blood picks up oxygen, then the other side pushes
the blood through the arms, legs, muscles, intestines, liver, and
brain. The heart is an electrically controlled pump. It has its own
internal electrical system, its own little brain, that governs how hard
and how often it contracts, or beats. It also receives governing nerve
impulses from the brain.

The whole system of internal pipes that carry the blood also has
its own electrical governing system. This system includes the
arteries, which contain the oxygen-full blood that is delivered out
into the body, and the veins, containing the oxygen-poor blood that
comes back to the lungs to be recharged. The size of these blood

vessels is controlled by the sympathetic and parasympathetic nervous systems, which in turn, are controlled mostly by the brain. These two nervous systems determine to what extent the blood vessels, the arteries in particular, are mostly open or mostly constricted. When the arteries are constricted and the heart beats very hard it produces an increase in the pressure of the blood. If this is a continuous condition it is known as high blood pressure, or "hypertension." If the heart beats very lightly and the blood vessels are mostly open you may have low blood pressure. If you have severe low blood pressure you might faint if you are standing up because there isn't enough pressure to get the blood all the way up to your brain. If the heart is beating regularly and the blood vessels are in a proper state of constriction, then the cardiovascular system is working perfectly satisfactorily.

The other thing you need to understand is that the heart muscle itself has its own arteries that provide the oxygen and other nourishment it needs to keep working. These are the "coronary" arteries.

▶▶ SOME KINDS OF HEART TROUBLE

These coronary arteries sometimes get hardened and partially plugged up as people get older. When the coronary arteries get too narrow to let enough blood go through, people often start having pain in the chest with exercise or strong emotion. This pain is called "angina pectoris," which, in Latin, simply means "pain in the chest." In effect, the pain signals that the muscles in the heart are not getting enough oxygen and so they start hurting. People who have angina pectoris, or simply "angina," usually get attacks when they exercise too much, get very upset or experience any other kind of strain that makes the heart beat faster and work harder.

Although I don't want you to diagnose your own condition at home without seeing a doctor, it may be helpful to point out what happens when the heart gets weak and a person has heart failure. If the left side of the heart begins to weaken but the right side of the heart is functioning all right, then the right side keeps pumping blood into the lungs faster than the left side can pump it out into the rest of the body. When this happens fluid and blood accumulate in the lungs. The lungs become swollen and congested and the person begins to have trouble breathing. With left-sided heart failure, then, an early sign of trouble is shortness of breath. This sometimes is most apparent when the individual lies down in bed. He may have trouble sleeping unless he is propped up on three, four, or five pillows. People sometimes also get acute attacks of shortness of breath in the middle of the night. People with trouble breathing due to heart problems get short of breath climbing even one flight of stairs. Any of these symptoms certainly make an immediate trip to the doctor highly desirable.

If the right side of the heart begins to fail first, then it will not pump blood out of the veins and into the lungs fast enough. Fluid and blood then back up in the body. This often leads to fluid being squeezed out of the smallest blood vessels. This is caused by the increased blood pressure in the veins due to the congestion in the right side of the heart. Fluid can leak out into body tissues, causing swollen ankles and, in more severe cases, swollen legs and even swollen abdomens. This is called "edema"; it used to be called, colloquially, "dropsy." As I described in the chapter on diuretics, edema can be caused by many things other than heart failure, but heart trouble can be one important cause.

It is also worth mentioning some conditions that seem to bother lay people a lot more than they bother doctors. Low blood pressure (hypotension) is often a cause of worry for some people. There are a few rare conditions in which blood pressure really is so low that people get dizzy and pass out. Then medical treatment is needed. However, merely having a relatively low set of numbers when blood pressure is taken, like 90/60, is not a cause for concern if you feel perfectly comfortable and can do all the normal activities of daily life without fainting or feeling dizzy every time you stand up. With abnormally low blood pressure, such as would be seen after a bad automobile accident or a severe injury of some sort, people are severely and obviously sick. They may be unconscious. Then, the low blood pressure requires immediate and urgent medical treatment. Most people who worry about low blood pressure are probably not seriously ill at all.

Some people also worry about getting short of breath. As I said before, shortness of breath can be caused by heart trouble of various sorts, but a lot of people get short of breath simply because they are out of condition. If you lead a very inactive life, do very little work, and are called upon to climb four flights of stairs, you are likely to get very short of breath, particularly if you are overweight, even if your heart is in perfectly good condition. People who jog a lot, on the other hand, can probably climb four flights of stairs without much difficulty. You must think about the possibility of heart trouble when there is shortness of breath, but most often it is determined by the physical condition, not by the presence of heart or lung disease.

I've also noticed that almost everybody, at one time or another, has been told that he has a heart "murmur." Lots of murmurs appear to be "functional," meaning there is no apparent cause and the doctor doesn't think it has any particularly ominous significance. Many people worry about their hearts because of a casual remark made by a doctor, in passing, that the doctor didn't think was important. However, the patient may get very upset and worry about it. Better doctor-patient relationships, finding a doctor in whom you can have real trust and whom you feel free to ask questions, is probably the best solution.

A lot of people's hearts will skip a beat from time to time. These missed beats are often not even noticed by the person, but sometimes they cause a sort of "flip-flop" sensation in the chest. This occurs particularly when lying in bed at night, worrying slightly about your heart or if your heart is pounding for some reason and you think about it. If you're busy doing something, like carrying on a conversation or doing some work, the skipped beat probably wouldn't even be noticed. These skipped beats usually come from "extra systoles," a technical word for extra beats. The extra systole can come from a single irritable point in a part of the heart. They are usually relatively benign though doctors may worry slightly if they are too frequent or if they originate in certain parts of the heart. These extra beats usually mean little or nothing. They may be aided and abetted by drinking too much coffee, smoking too many cigarettes, or getting too anxious and upset. If you are bothered by them, of course, you should consult your doctor, but if you can't see him right away — and it's not usually an emergency situation — you might try cutting down on your coffee intake and stop smoking to see whether that will make it go away. The chemicals in coffee and cigarettes tend to make the heart more excitable.

There are abnormal conditions in which a person's heart rhythm goes all to pieces and his heart bumps along totally irregularly. This rhythm is usually known as "auricular fibrillation" and is most often found in people having some underlying form of heart disease such as rheumatic fever or hardening of the arteries. However, it can be aggravated by an overactive thyroid gland.

The heart can beat very rapidly for other reasons also. It is usually thought that resting rates under one hundred twenty beats a minute are not particularly remarkable. High rates occur with states of anxiety, a high fever, or after a lot of exercise. I've had heart rates of over two hundred beats per minute during extremely heavy exertion. People who have a resting heart rate of one hundred fifty to one hundred seventy beats per minute are usually short of breath and in some cardiac distress. This is known as "auricular tachycardia" or, much more rarely, "ventricular tachycardia." This is an emergency. It requires medical treatment at the nearest emergency room or an immediate call to your doctor.

Digitalis and Related Drugs

The digitalis group of drugs is probably the most effective and most impressive set of cardiovascular agents in existence. It is the drug most often used to strengthen the heart in failure, that is, when either one or both sides of the heart aren't pumping hard enough. It is historically interesting to note that an ancient Chinese remedy consisting of dried toad skin was probably an effective agent for a failing heart because it contained a digitalis-like chemical. In Western medicine, digitalis was used by ancient Welsh physicians as an extract of foxglove, a common flower. The "digit-" part of digitalis means "finger" in Latin. The formal botanical name of foxglove is *Digitalis purpurea* because the flower resembles a purple finger. The most famous paper on digitalis, "An Account of the Foxglove and Some of Its Medical Uses with Practical Remarks on Dropsy and Other Diseases," was published as early as 1785 by William Withering. It is still a classic example of careful clinical observation of a drug's use in medicine. As I mentioned before, "dropsy" used to be the term for all kinds of things causing swelling of the limbs — edema of the ankles and other parts of the body. Withering observed that digitalis helped in some cases of dropsy but not in others. Medicine was too primitive at that point for him to discriminate between heart trouble and kidney trouble. He thought the drug worked on the kidneys since it caused people to pass a lot of water and thus get rid of their edema or "dropsy." He was wrong as to the specific mechanism of action. On the other hand, he was very accurate in describing how to use the drug, its side effects, and its main effects.

The main action of digitalis is to increase the strength of each heartbeat. When the heart is weakened by bad valves, hardening of the arteries, or chronic high blood pressure, digitalis will enable it to beat harder and, thereby, pump more blood. Often, this increased pumping action will cure the backing up of blood that causes edema in the lungs or in the lower extremities. Digitalis literally makes the heart muscle squeeze harder. Digitalis has a lot of other effects on the heart but these effects are far more complicated and of less importance than its effect of strengthening heart action and relieving chronic heart failure.

It is not a very safe drug. Its lethal dose is probably not much more than two to three times the dose at which people begin to get results. Nevertheless, the drug is so remarkable in its effect that it is well worth using under careful medical supervision. It can be dangerous if improperly used. It is clearly a drug that should be taken only with the direction and close supervision of a physician while an appropriate daily dose is being worked out. People who have chronic heart failure can take appropriate amounts of digitalis daily for a long time without getting into trouble at all.

The early side effects of digitalis and related drugs include nausea, vomiting, and diarrhea. Interestingly, at somewhat more toxic doses, patients' vision may be tinged yellow or green or they may have facial pain for unknown pharmacological reasons. The drug may also cause the heart to develop extra systoles and can change the rhythm and rate of the heartbeat. Digitalis-like drugs and their usual oral doses are: digitalis powder, digitalis tablets, or digitalis at 0.06 mg to 1 gm; ouabain (Strophanthin-G) injected as needed; digitoxin 0.05 mg to 0.25 mg; digoxin (Lanoxin) 0.25 to 0.5 mg; lanatoside C 0.5 mg (Cedilanid); deslanoside (Cedilanid-D) injected as needed; acetyldigitoxin (Acylanid) 0.1 to 0.2 mg; and gitalin (Gitaligin) 0.5 mg.

As I noted in the chapter on diuretics, drugs such as chlorothiazide are often used along with drugs of the digitalis class in the treatment of chronic heart failure. They can do a great deal to keep patients free of edema, comfortable, and active when they would otherwise be in substantial distress.

Antiarrhythmic Drugs

Several drugs are used to stop abnormal heart rhythms. Digitalis, for many years, was thought to be effective for patients who had auricular fibrillation. Although digitalis slowed the beating of the heart in people who had rapid, irregular heart action due to auricular fibrillation, its main effect really was in increasing the efficiency of individual heartbeats. This slowed the heart rate, even though it did not directly adjust the heart rhythm. Digitalis ordinarily will not correct the heart rhythm from an abnormal to a normal one. Quinidine (Quinamin) is effective in slowing rapid heart rates and in converting, in some cases, auricular fibrillation to a steady, normal rate. Unfortunately, this drug can also be somewhat toxic. It can cause side effects similar to those of aspirin overdose. Also, since quinidine works directly on the heart muscle to make it less excitable, the dose that causes the heart muscle to work more slowly and regularly is relatively close to the dose that can cause more serious effects.

Another group of drugs that control the rhythmicity of the heart is typified by propranolol (Inderal). This type of drug works by blocking the nerves that act to cause the heart to speed up due to exercise or emotion. At a usual dose of 10 mg to 40 mg, it differs from quinidine in that it acts mostly on the nervous input to the heart whereas quinidine works on the heart itself. The end effect, however, is much the same — a slower, more regular heartbeat. Another drug that acts somewhat like propranolol is diphenylhydantoin (Dilantin), the anticonvulsive agent already discussed. Treatment with drugs of this sort should be closely monitored by a physician and should never be embarked on independently by a patient.

Coronary Vasodilators

As I mentioned earlier in this chapter, some people develop a severe, crushing, and extraordinarily unpleasant pain in the region of the chest with severe or, in more serious cases, mild exertion or emotion. This is the pain of angina pectoris. It originates in heart muscle that is not getting enough oxygen to enable it to do the work that the body systems are telling it to do. This increased need by the heart for oxygen can be treated. At the present time, the commonest and safest drugs used for treatment are relatively short acting. They are organic nitrites. Amyl nitrite is available as little pearl-like capsules that are crushed and inhaled. This drug is absorbed through the nasal mucous membrane and causes a rapid and immediate dilation of the arteries of the heart, thereby increasing the oxygen supply to heart muscle, which relieves the pain. Nitroglycerin (Nitrol) — the same chemical that is used as an explosive — is given, 0.2 mg to 0.6 mg, as sublingual tablets. Sublingual means "under the tongue." You take the tablet or lozenge by keeping it under your tongue and waiting for it to be absorbed. It is given that way because it is absorbed faster through the mucous membranes of the mouth than it would be if swallowed as a pill. Since angina comes on suddenly and quite painfully, the drug must get into the bloodstream as rapidly as possible. That's the reason why the two most commonly used drugs for this condition are given by such unusual routes. Other similar drugs are: sodium nitrite at 30 mg to 60 mg, erythrityl tetranitrate (Cardilate) at 5 mg to 15 mg, pentaerythitol tetranitrate (Peritrate and others) at 10 mg to 30 mg, isosorbide dinitrate (Isordil) at 10 mg to 40 mg, mannitol hexanitrate, and trolnitrate phosphate at 8 mg to 40 mg.

Nitroglycerin is longer acting than amyl nitrite. Its effects may last as long as a half hour and, to a limited extent, it can be given prophylactically, that is, someone with angina pectoris can take it before he is about to do something that would ordinarily give him an attack of angina to prevent the attack. This enables him to lead a fairly normal life. As of this writing, I am aware of no long-acting drug that has been medically proven to prevent angina. From time to time drugs are developed that are supposed to have this action, but it is too early to be sure of any of them. If you have angina, perhaps a consultation with your internist (a specialist in internal medicine) or cardiologist (a heart specialist) will give you the opportunity to try one of the newer, investigational drugs that *may* have such an effect. Obviously, a drug that would avert all angina in a patient suffering from this painful and frightening illness would be a great blessing.

Antihypertensive Agents

Antihypertensive means "against high blood pressure." There are a fairly large number of drugs and a variety of different classes of drugs that may help reduce high blood pressure. Fortunately, some cases of mild high blood pressure can be brought under control without drugs. In fact, your blood pressure tends to go up if you are tense, jumpy, or scared. For example, if you are seeing a new doctor or, perhaps, even if told you might have high blood pressure, you could become tense enough to raise your blood pressure to a level high enough for it to be considered abnormal. Just getting used to your doctor, the examining room, and the whole situation might bring your blood pressure back to normal without any drugs at all. As a test to find out how really severe a blood pressure problem might be, doctors used to give patients barbiturates to see whether their blood pressure would come down when they were asleep. If the pressure went down, this was an indication that it was *labile,* a term meaning that it goes up or down depending on the patient's situation; it is not always high. Sometimes if people lose weight their hearts don't have to work so hard and their blood pressure may drop for that reason alone.

If blood pressure is too high — and it can be a serious life-threatening illness when it gets very high and stays that way for prolonged periods — doctors will use various drugs to treat it. The two classes of drugs probably most commonly used in mild high blood pressure, that is, high blood pressure that is just a bit over the 140/90 threshold, are diuretics of the benzothiadiazide type, such as chlorothiazide (Diuril), or drugs like reserpine (Serpasil). As far as I can determine, no one really knows why chlorothiazide lowers people's blood pressure. It does so even when people have no edema and the kidneys do not put out any more water than usual.

The effect on blood pressure, therefore, appears to be completely independent of the action on excretion and is, as far as I am concerned, a complete mystery.

The action of reserpine-like drugs is probably tied to their effect on hormones in the nerves that play a role in the transmission of nerve impulses. These neural hormones are particularly important in the sympathetic nervous system where norepinephrine has a specific role in making blood vessel muscles contract. One cause of high blood pressure is tight blood vessels. This might be due to the presence of too much norepinephrine. Reserpine has the property of making the nerve endings let go of norepinephrine, and this tends to reduce blood pressure. Unfortunately, the drug also makes people drowsy. It is a modestly effective major tranquilizer. It also tends to give people stuffy noses, nausea, and a wide range of mildly unpleasant side effects that make it a less pleasant drug for a patient to take than one of the chlorothiazide-like drugs. These two drugs are sometimes given together if one of them alone does not help.

For more severe hypertension, a drug somewhat similar to reserpine is used, called methyldopa (Aldomet). This drug takes the place of norepinephrine and similar neural hormones at the nerve endings. It deceives the nerve endings in the same way that sulfa drugs deceive germs. It looks like norepinephrine but doesn't act like it, so it makes the blood vessels relax. Both methyldopa and reserpine have other complex effects in brain centers that probably have something to do with the control of blood pressure as well. Methyldopa will work for some patients who have high blood pressure when reserpine does not.

Another drug that works on the neural hormones is pargyline (Eutonyl). This drug decreases the destruction of norepinephrine and similar chemicals at the nerve endings. Although pargyline has this effect on neural hormones it is by no means clear that pargyline's ability to lower blood pressure is related to this pharmacological property since the antihypertensive effect comes on rather slowly and appears to be independent of the degree of effect on norepinephrine.

Another drug, hydralazine (Apresoline), appears to work by having a direct relaxing effect on muscles and arteries in the body. The mechanism by which it has its effect is quite unclear. Its side effects include headache, palpitation, nausea, vomiting, and diarrhea. It may also cause constipation and difficulty in passing water. In general, this drug is thought to be less useful than the others mentioned. Doctors have varying ideas about it, and the evidence concerning its utility is sufficiently mixed that one must trust the doctor's judgment and his past experience with it.

Guanethidine (Ismelin) is said to be the mainstay of the management of severe hypertension, but its use is rare enough that it may well be outside the scope of this book. It has a direct paralyzing effect on the nerve impulses going to the blood vessels that cause vessel constriction. Therefore, a direct blocking effect of high blood pressure is obtained. It probably works too well. Patients maintained on guanethidine do not have high blood pressure, but their blood pressure regulating system is also somewhat paralyzed. They may get dizzy or pass out when they rise from a lying to a sitting position and their whole cardiovascular system may not react at all normally to the increase in vessel size required by exercise. Patients may find that this drug severely limits their activities and produces rather unpleasant side effects. People taking this drug often feel generally weak. Some people using it develop edema because blood isn't pumped through the body quite as efficiently. Some people develop diarrhea, and the drug not uncommonly interferes with ejaculation in the male. This may develop further into an impotence, a complication less likely to be directly due to the drug than to a psychological effect caused by the failure of ejaculation.

Despite its unpleasant side effects guanethidine appears to be the most effective agent available for treatment of severe hypertension. Severe hypertension is a dangerous condition that may lead to strokes or to heart attacks.

The different drugs that are used in various medical conditions affecting the heart are complicated. Often their margin of safety is not particularly large and their side effects tend to be unpleasant. They obviously are not drugs that should be traded from person to person, given to one's friends or taken lightly as self-medication for imagined heart ailments. If you believe you have a heart condition you certainly should get competent medical advice and assistance. If you have a chronic and serious heart condition you should follow your doctor's advice closely. However, the material presented in this chapter may help you formulate questions that you may wish to discuss with your doctor about your individual difficulties. I hope it may lead to a better understanding of the usefulness of the drugs you are taking and the ways in which they should be taken. Although I have often not gone into detailed discussions of duration of action and dosage, these are every bit as important and probably more important with cardiovascular drugs than they are with other drugs such as aspirin. Therefore, it is important to discuss with your doctor the effects you get, their relation to the time you take your medication, whether you should take your medication before or after meals, the kinds of side effects you may be getting or believe you're getting, and other similar issues. Obviously, anyone with a chronic heart condition is likely not to feel very good some of the time. It is necessary to find out the difference between possible drug side effects and the symptoms of the illness.

It is also worth noting that the drug treatments now available for heart failure, high blood pressure, heart rhythm irregularities, and angina pectoris are substantial improvements over what medicine could offer even fifty years ago. Current research seems to be coming up with even more useful drugs for the various cardiovascular conditions.

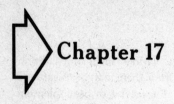

Chapter 17

Hallucinogens and Marijuana

In every culture, throughout the recorded history of mankind, people have consumed herbs, plants, beverages, or even certain types of fish in order to obtain a mental experience different from that found in their everyday lives. The earliest recorded history of the use of these mind-altering drugs was in 2000 B.C. A group of tribes known as Aryans resided in an area extending from parts of Russia through Finland. These Aryan tribes began a migration south into Europe, through Asia Minor, finally crossing into India. Here the Aryans waged war on the natives of ancient India called the Dravidians. They won this encounter and so took over the rule of India. From the poems and religious writings of these Aryan tribes we have an account of the use of the drug soma. Soma occupied a central place in the religion of these people. A large number of the verses in the Rig-Veda, the most ancient of religious writings, are paeans of exultation to soma and the mental state it would produce. For many years scholars have wondered what the plant referred to in the Rig-Veda might be that could confer upon people so many marvelous experiences. One interesting aspect of the pharmacology of this substance led to the discovery of the specific plant. The Rig-Veda stated that after the ingestion of the plant by the holy men of the tribe, they would then urinate and the congregation would drink their urine so that they also might experience the ecstatic state. Recently, predominantly through the efforts of Gordon Wasson, the drug soma has been identified as the product of the mushroom *Amanita muscaria*. Four thousand years later we have found a plant that contains a hallucinogenic substance that can be ingested and excreted in an almost unchanged form in the urine.

Another example of the building of a religion around the ritual use of a chemical substance that has the property to alter one's mental state comes from this hemisphere. South American Indians, from the most primitive tribes of the Amazon to the highly developed, cultured Aztecs, all used various forms of chemical substances obtained from plants to achieve a change of mental state. The Aztecs, particularly, had a series of such substances that they called "magic" or "witch" drugs. Lately, we have managed to identify some of these drugs. One is the Aztec witch drug, ololiuqui, which is made from the seeds of a particular type of morning glory. This substance has been found to contain lysergic acid amide. This chemical is a close relative of lysergic acid diethylamide (LSD, acid). Ololiuqui was used in holy rituals to attain a trance state so that the priests could advise the chiefs of the Aztec nation as to the views of the gods on the proper ways to guide their people.

Some of the less developed tribes of South America, such as the Waika Indians, still use substances to change their view of the world. Many of these chemicals are taken as a snuff that is blown up the nose of the user. Most of these snuffs contain harmine, alkaloids that are related to other known hallucinogenic chemicals. In these tribes the use of hallucinogenic drugs is not formal or ritualized. It seems to be something that people do whenever they want to. The reason these tribes use the snuff can perhaps be best summarized by the actual statement of one of the Waika Indians when asked why he used it. He stated that the use of the snuff made him "tall enough to speak to his gods." So, though not ritualized or formalized as in some of the other tribes, the use of these mind-altering chemicals still has a religious context. The user tries to experience some type of ecstatic state that makes him feel more perceptive of or receptive to the will of the gods. This is similar to many statements made by modern American hallucinogen users when asked why they use this type of drug.

In the South Seas, other drugs have been used that are hallucinogenic. One of the major drugs used in the Polynesian group is called kava. If one grinds the fresh plant, one can produce a brew of kava that is such a stimulant it will produce incoordination and cause changes in the way the user sees the world. Kava in a different form is still used by these island groups. It is the ritual welcome drink of the islands. When President and Mrs. Johnson went to the American Samoan Islands, they were given a traditional sip of kava. The present form is made from dried kava. It does not possess hallucinogenic properties. It is merely a mildly stimulating drink, more or less like a cup of coffee.

Many other examples could be described from different cultures at different times in world history to show that man has an abiding need, occasionally, to seek alternate ways of viewing his world and his life. Generally, these needs have been associated with religious rituals. The use of these drugs seems to facilitate man's sense of the infinite, of God, and of his own relationship to other men and to his universe. Perhaps these brief examples from history will help make the present use of hallucinogenic substances by some people a little less puzzling. These substances have always served as initiation rites for entry into some groups. They still do. They have always been what might be called an "emotional physical fitness" test that lets people try to prove their capacity by seeing just how far they can go and still come back. They have always fulfilled a need of man to have experiences that are different, new, and novel. Finally, they have always been used in a ritualistic, religious manner. Indeed, these drugs have very aptly been called "cultogenic" drugs. They are almost always used by individuals in small groups and their use tends to develop into religions or cults.

Undoubtedly, this is one of the more difficult subjects to discuss. At present, there is no approved medical therapeutic usage for the hallucinogenic chemicals. On the other hand, though not widespread, the drugs are present in our culture to a great enough extent that many people have heard about them and quite a few have experienced their effects. Perhaps 3 to 5 percent of college students have used one or more of the hallucinogenic drugs at one time or another. Further, quantities of sensationalistic publicity have come out about these drugs, both pro and con. They may be described as producing a beautiful, wonderful experience or as very dangerous drugs that will lead to chromosome damage and suicide. To balance these extremes, I will try to describe these chemicals in the same way that I would describe any other drug; the effects of the chemicals are going to depend upon the purity of the compounds, the amount you take, how often you take them, what your particular situation is, and what you expect the drugs to do for you.

Lysergic Acid Diethylamide (LSD)

Lysergic acid diethylamide was discovered by A. E. Hoffman in 1943. The story goes that Hoffman was working in his laboratory preparing a compound that had been developed from the chemical ergot, which is a natural product of a fungus disease of rye plants. A new form of the drug was being tested in the hope of finding a useful medicinal product. Apparently, Dr. Hoffman had sniffed and got some of the LSD into his lungs or onto his tongue at the wrong time — just a very tiny amount. Later, that afternoon, he reported that he had a dreamlike state and a feeling somewhat similar to drunkenness with an exaggerated imagination. Dr. Hoffman was not at all sure that this was due to the drug but he suspected it might be. So, the next day, he met with some of his colleagues and tried a small amount again. Sure enough, the effect had been due to the drug. Actually, Dr. Hoffman used a dose of 0.25 mg orally, thinking that would be a safe dose since it was quite low. The result was somewhat spectacular and we now know that he took five to ten times the amount that would have been necessary to produce mental changes in susceptible people.

The finding demonstrated that a chemical could cause significant changes in a susceptible person's perception of the world at a dose as low as 20 mcg to 25 mcg. This was an exceedingly important discovery for pharmacology. Until that time, we did not have information on any other drug that worked at so low a dose. Thus, everyone was quite excited about it. Further, the state produced by the drug was one in which people would laugh a lot, become emotional, sometimes cry, and would cycle in and out of emotional states with fear as well as happiness. Sometimes common objects would be experienced as particularly fascinating — crystals would shine more strongly, colors were much more intense and bright and there was marked distortion of the person's perception. Another characteristic experience caused by the drug is called "depersonalization." A person begins to lose his distinct sense of identity. Thus, he becomes more at one with his universe and his surroundings. He is not quite sure who he is or where he stops. His identity extends beyond his skin. Further, this same state can be characterized generally by feelings of religiosity, of having an ecstatic vision and a oneness with the universe. If you have lost the separateness of your specific identity from the rest of the universe, perhaps you are as one with everything else too.

This mental state resembles the way psychiatrists have described some mental disturbances called "psychoses." For this reason, some of these drugs have been called "psychotomimetics," that is, they mimic psychoses. However, most recent evidence has shown that this is really quite a different mental state from the psychotic condition. Rather, these drugs produce changes in mood, distortions in the way one perceives the world, and changes in one's feelings about the world. Particularly, these drugs cause an enhancement of visual sensation so things seem sharper and clearer, though quite often distorted. They do not produce auditory hallucinations, which are a common perceptual phenomena found in many of the psychoses. In all honesty, I have known very few people who have used these drugs who did not find the experience with this changed mental state intellectually and emotionally interesting — not always pleasant, but interesting. However, as with any very different experience, some people don't like it at all, and most people get bored with it after a few "trips."

The dose-response curve for lysergic acid diethylamide (LSD) has a threshold dose of 20 mcg to 25 mcg in a very susceptible individual by the oral route. Its effects increase to a ceiling dose of approximately 800 mcg. The therapeutic safety ratio is exceedingly high. We don't know exactly how high it is, since, to this time, no human being has been killed due to the acute toxic effects of an overdose of LSD. From animal studies, however, we would guess the therapeutic safety ratio to be somewhere in the neighborhood of 1:5,000 to 1:10,000. The time-action of lysergic acid has an onset of approximately ten to twenty minutes after the oral ingestion and a cessation of action about four to eight hours after it has been taken.

The mechanism of action of LSD is not known. There are some theories about it but they do not make enough sense at this time to be worth discussion here.

There are a number of adverse side effects associated with the use of LSD. However, let me make a few points very clear. First, LSD is rapidly tolerated. Within a few days, if one takes continual doses of this drug, it will cease to have any effectiveness. Therefore, one cannot stay on an LSD trip for over a couple of days or so, no matter how much drug he takes. Second, the usual pattern of drug taking is to use it only occasionally. The vast majority of people who have used LSD have taken it only from one to three times. Then, they never use it again in their lives. There have been some people who have taken LSD hundreds and indeed, thousands of times, but these are rare cases. Even then, they can stop whenever they wish.

The majority, well over 90 percent, have used the drug only a few times and then have no urge to continue to take the chemical. This demonstrates that not only is tolerance rapidly developed for the drug in acute use, but also no dependence, either psychological or physical, is developed by the majority of people, and no person develops physical dependence even with prolonged use.

Many people have wondered about the long-term effects of the use of LSD. It appears at this time that there are no long-term effects from a few episodes of use of LSD. Studies have been performed on over five thousand volunteer subjects who received this drug in experimental circumstances. Followups of these people for a number of years have shown them to be no different from other people of similar age group and type, in either health or social activity. It did not harm them to have a few exposures in an experimental setting.

Another adverse effect following the use of LSD that has often been reported is suicide. Until 1967, and this is the latest date for which we have documentation, there were only eleven cases of proven and documented suicide by persons while under the influence of LSD. Probably by now, there are twenty or fewer proven suicide cases. These cases have probably been reported a thousand times each. But all the different reports are related to the same few proven cases. Two things may have led to this over-reporting of suicide due to LSD. First, it might not be realized that adolescents are the second most likely group of persons to commit suicide. Indeed, the number of adolescent suicides has gone up almost 200 percent in the last ten years. This proneness to suicide is true as well for members of this age group who don't use drugs. Second, during recovery from an LSD experience people will often have thoughts of suicide that they report to others. Few actually ever attempt suicide but they do talk about it. These two facts may have led to the general belief that the drug causes suicide. This seems not to be the case. In the vast majority of cases we have no evidence that LSD has a high suicide potential. Certainly, when one compares it with drugs like alcohol, barbiturates, or aspirin, it is one of the minor causes of drug-produced suicide in the United States today.

Another subject that has led to vast speculation and apprehension is the so-called flashback phenomenon. First, it seems that flashback occurs in fewer than 1 percent of the cases in which LSD has been used. Second, the flashback experience can continue for an hour or so but, in most of the cases, lasts only a few seconds. Third, the flashback experience, if it is going to, will happen in the first year after the use of LSD.

Flashback is a very difficult phenomenon to understand or explain. Certainly there is no rational reason to believe that it is directly due to any drug left in your body. A more psychological explanation is probably best. One theory, and I stress it is only a theory, but one that makes sense to me, is that flashback is a psychological phenomenon in which a small part of your immediate environment can call back to your present experience the whole of a previous, very dramatic situation. This happens to all of us. Perhaps the best known cases have been reported by soldiers who have seen combat. Combat is a very dramatic, different experience for a person. At a later date, when a soldier is not in combat, some very small aspect of his environment, for example, a siren, might all of a sudden cause him to break out in a cold sweat and dive under his desk. Thus, a small part of his environment makes him suddenly relive the very dramatic experience that he previously had in combat. All of us can, at one time or another, have all of the emotion and much of the experience of a dramatic incident come back, all of a sudden, for no obvious reason. This may be what is happening in flashbacks. The person has had a very dramatic and different experience while under the influence of LSD. At a later time, a small stimulus in his environment can cause a full, emotional repeat of the LSD experience. This usually lasts for only a few seconds, but may last for a period of time. Whether this is, or is not, the explanation for flashback I don't know. But, as I said, this is the theory that makes the most sense to me.

Another highly publicized phenomenon said to be associated with LSD use is the production of malformed babies. This must be carefully defined since it is really two different subjects. First, there is the subject called the teratological effects of a drug. This is what the drug might do when taken by a pregnant woman. Thalidomide has a teratological effect. The second question is, Does the drug produce damage to the chromosomes in egg or sperm cells in the person who uses the drug? This is a genetic question. Some initial evidence showed that LSD might possibly cause genetic damage. Since this first evidence, the drug has been studied many times by very good scientists. At this time, there is no evidence that any greater damage is caused to chromosomes in one's eggs or sperm by LSD than could be caused by aspirin. The consideration, Does LSD cause problems if it is taken by a pregnant woman? is not quite as certain. There have been studies that have suggested that possibly, in pregnant rats, if the drug is taken just before the rat pups are born, there may be some stunting of growth and some greater likelihood of abnormalities. However, in studies on humans who have taken not only LSD but also vast numbers of other kinds of drugs as well, this has not been confirmed. At this time, we have no evidence that the taking of LSD by a pregnant human female will cause a greater likelihood of the development of a birth defect in the child. Note that I added to both statements the cautious phrase, we have no evidence. That doesn't mean that more evidence can't be obtained in the future that will show some effects. On the other hand, this chance of the discovery of some new problem is a possibility with every drug. We always worry about this happening. But, at this time, we don't have any reason to believe that LSD is any more dangerous in causing genetic or teratological effects than any other drug.

Another problem with LSD is the development of mental difficulties in a few people who were on the borderline of mental illness beforehand. When these people take the drug they can flip out. Of the possibly 1 to 3 percent of all people who do take LSD there may be a few who will not have enough mental stability to recover quickly from the effects of the drug. These people become agitated and confused, and have a mental state that resembles a psychosis. The majority of these people, between 50 and 70 percent of those who have this particular problem due to taking LSD, if admitted to psychiatric care will be well enough to go home within forty-eight hours. However, a certain percentage, perhaps 30 percent, of those who get this mental agitation will have to stay in the hospital six months or longer. This particular result is one of the hazards of the drug. You will note that it doesn't happen to everyone who takes LSD. It seems to happen to only a relatively small percent of all users, and most of those affected get better quickly. Another way of saying this is that our mental hospitals are not filled up with people who have freaked out on LSD. Some professionals have even proposed that this is a very good way to find disturbed people in order to help them. However, this is not a proposal that has been widely accepted, since some of the long lasting mental disturbances caused by LSD do not respond well to psychiatric treatment.

The final problem that emerges when discussing LSD is the fact that people who obtain the drug on the street really don't know what they are getting. Usually, it was made by clandestine laboratories. The buyer does not know the purity of the substance. He does not even know whether it is really LSD. Also, he doesn't know the dose he receives. This certainly is a problem. It's difficult to talk about drugs when you can't be sure precisely what you have taken, how pure it was, or how much was taken. As an example, of seventy-five samples that were purchased on the streets of San Francisco, all of which were sold as LSD, only three actually had any LSD in them. The others contained all sorts of strange chemicals that were difficult to identify — but they weren't LSD. The street buyer may be receiving a rather poisonous mixture, at doses that he doesn't know. He could be in a very dangerous position. As an example, some LSD samples on the street today contain strychnine. At even relatively low doses, strychnine can kill. The idea is that the user first has a strychnine convulsion, then, as he is recovering from the convulsion, which is very unpleasant, in fact hair-raising, he goes into the pleasure of the LSD state. Supposedly, the terror of the convulsion makes the LSD an even greater pleasure. I think I'll find my kicks some other way. This doesn't appeal to me.

Another factor that must be taken into consideration is the expectation of the experience. The use of LSD is primarily a group activity. Generally, at least one person in the group, who is often called the "guide," is experienced. The guide sets the group expectation. He usually doesn't take the drug but takes care of the rest of the group. If a drug is taken with the expectation of a good, smooth trip, if the room is pleasant and has pleasant things to look at, there is pleasant music, and there are people around you love, trust, and feel kinship for, the odds are that you will have a good trip — a pleasant experience for the most part. Even under ideal conditions, however, there may still be periods in which you begin to panic a little. But if there's someone there to reassure you, to help you roll with the drug, and if you have adequate mental stability, you will probably have an interesting experience. The effects will come in waves. There may be periods of panic and anxiety, but, for the most part, it will be a pleasant experience. On the other hand, if you do not have the mental stability, if you don't have the correct preparation and don't know what to expect from the drug, you're uptight, a bit anxious and afraid about taking it, you're not sure that you trust the people in your room, or you're alone and have a lot on your mind, your chances of having a very unpleasant experience, perhaps a real "bummer," are fairly high. The drug creates a mind opened to the influences in the environment. The expectations of the person and his environment, to a large extent, will determine the precise nature of the drug trip.

Mescaline

Mescaline is the chemical that is the active constituent of the button found on the top of a mature cactus plant named peyote or peyotl. It has been used for centuries, before the white man ever came to this continent, by American Indian tribes, particularly those of the northern Mexican area. Indeed, our first information about this hallucinogen came from the writings of the Franciscan monk Bernardino de Sahagún in 1560. During the Spanish Conquest of Mexico, the Catholic church was very much against the use of the peyote cactus, since it was used as part of the Indian religious worship. Part of the missionary work of the Spaniards was to attempt to stamp out the use of this plant around which much of the native religion centered.

Later, in 1918, Indians in the United States began to use this plant as part of their worship services. They organized its use into a formal religion now called the Native American Church of North America. This church still exists. It has members from all the Indian tribes across the United States. Part of the ritual of the Native American Church is the eating of the peyote button to obtain the blessings, healing powers, and understanding of the Great Spirit. This is a perfectly legal use of the drug. The Supreme Court has ruled that this use of peyote is not an affront to the law or to society. The legal use of peyote is permitted only to members of the Native American Church.

At the present time, pure mescaline is obtained by chemical synthesis as well as from an extract of peyote. It is sold illegally on the streets. "Street" mescaline is of a notoriously low quality with many impurities.

Mescaline is a close relative of the stimulant amphetamine, as are a number of other hallucinogenic compounds. Other hallucinogenic compounds of the amphetamine-like series have a subjective effect similar to that of mescaline. However, other chemicals of this type differ in the dose necessary to achieve an effect and, also, the length of time that they act. Some of these are, trimethoxy-amphetamine (TMA), dimethoxyamphetamine (DMA), methylene-dioxyamphetamine (MDA), methoxymethyleneoxyamphetamine (MMDA), dimethoxymethyleneoxyamphetamine (DMMDA), methoxyamphetamine (MA), dimethoxymethylamphetamine (DOM, Serenity, Tranquility, Peace, STP), and dimethoxyethylamphetamine (DOEP). Since all of these drugs are more similar than they are different, I will discuss them all together.

If one eats between six to twelve buttons of the peyote cactus, the usual first response for most people is to vomit. Some people have so much difficulty keeping this material down that they never do experience any of the mental effects caused by the drug. However, for those who do manage to hold enough of the material down, some rather dramatic effects are experienced. These effects are similar to, but in some ways different from, those observed with lysergic acid diethylamide. In a way similar to LSD, the drug causes perceptual distortion, heightened sense of color, enhanced self-awareness, some depersonalization, and a state of heightened mood. Mescaline experiences seem to differ from those of LSD in that the color and perceptual phenomena are more vivid under mescaline than under LSD. Also, there seem to be very few bad trips on mescaline. For the most part, one's mood is up and there are very few panic reactions. This is, of course, particularly true when it is taken as part of the ceremony of the North American Church. In this case, the user is expecting a beneficial effect, he is surrounded by a religious atmosphere, and the drug is taken with the support of the rest of the group. Its use is within a cultural tradition. All these factors favor a pleasant, useful, and interesting experience.

The usual dose of pure mescaline necessary to produce such an experience is approximately 350 mg to 500 mg. It is not as potent a drug as LSD; it takes a great deal more mescaline to get an effect. Generally, the onset of mescaline action is quite delayed; two to four hours is about the usual time before a strong experience starts. The mescaline experience tends to last longer than the LSD effect — perhaps twelve hours, on the average, before all vestiges of the experience have passed. All the other drugs of this series, particularly DOM, are more potent than mescaline. An adequate dose of DOM is 10 mg. With this large a dose, the effect can last quite a long time, up to sixteen to twenty-four hours. With this long an effect the person can have panic reactions — a very bad trip. Thus, the duration and intensity of the effect caused by high doses of these drugs seem to combine to cause more unpleasant reactions than are usually found with moderate doses of pure mescaline or peyote.

Tryptamines

Another group of hallucinogenic drugs, which also closely resemble lysergic acid diethylamide in their action, are psilocybin, psilocin, bufotenine, dimethyltriptamine (DMT), diethyltriptamine (DET), and harmine. The desired subjective effects and undesired effects of these compounds are essentially identical with those of LSD. These chemicals have a very interesting history. They have been used by various Indian tribes in Central America and Mexico for many years. Psilocybin, bufotenine, and psilocin are obtained from mushrooms in this area. The harmine-type drugs can be found in all manner of shrubs and plants in South America. In South America, harmine-containing plants are used by the natives either as snuff or as drinks. They are called by such names as Cappi or Yaje.

All of these drugs have a much lower potency than LSD. For example, with psilocybin or psilocin it takes about 48 mg to get any LSD-like effects. With DET or DMT the necessary dose ranges up to 150 mg to obtain the effect. Another difference in the effects of DMT and DET from the effects of LSD is their time of action. The effects upon ingestion will last, from an onset of three to four minutes, for about one hour. For this reason, since they are such short acting compounds with only an hour as a time-action, they have been called drugs for a "businessman's trip." You can trip out at lunch time and still get back to work in the afternoon.

The South American drinks or snuffs containing harmine have a different nature. Their onset is characterized by vomiting, convulsions, and tremor, followed by a ritual prancing dance that lasts from thirty minutes to two hours. Then, the user falls down into a deep sleep. To obtain this effect if the drugs had been given subcutaneously, it would require a dose somewhere betwen 125 mg and 200 mg.

Harmine-type drugs differ in other ways from LSD. Although we have not yet had any reports of human deaths, these drugs do not have the high therapeutic safety ratio that LSD, mescaline, DET, DMT, psilocybin, and psilocin do. It appears that the therapeutic safety ratio may be about 1:5. Also the reports on the nature of the subjective experiences caused by the harmine-type drugs differ from those of LSD. With the harmine there is a feeling of nausea, dizziness, and tiredness. The user loses sensation in his hands and feet. His body becomes numb. Also, before the depersonalization takes place between one's self and the objects of one's environment, there is not the experience of a heightened color sense.

The final group of hallucinogens to be discussed is typified by the drug phencyclidine (Sernyl, Hog, PCP). This chemical was first developed for use in veterinary medicine. It is presently used as an analgesic for animals. Also, a close analog of it, cyclohexamine (Ketamine), is presently being used in certain types of human operations as an analgesic and anesthetic to change the state of consciousness of a patient without producing a loss of consciousness or lowering of respiration as anesthetics generally do. These types of drugs are called "dissociative" agents. They use the property of causing a person to feel separated from his body to minimize the traumatic experience of a surgical operation.

Doses of phencyclidine in the range of 3 mg to 5 mg cause depersonalization. At this dose, by the intravenous route, the person will have a rapid heart rate, various kinds of mental dysfunctions, sweating, excessive salivation, some motor incoordination, a loss of deep pain sensation, and, possibly later, a loss of consciousness. The person experiences a feeling of depersonalization in which his mind floats away from his body and drifts freely in space. It is this characteristic that makes the drug a valuable adjunct in removing some of the trauma of pain in surgical operations. Sometimes, after the use of this chemical, which acts for about two hours, there can be a severe sense of apathy and lack of energy.

In one way phencyclidine is quite different from the other hallucinogens we have discussed. In a study in which fifty-five patients were given phencyclidine, only three of them laughed or reported any happiness. The rest were overwhelmed with fright and unpleasant experiences. Most people never wanted to take the drug again. I wonder why a drug of this nature is used illegally at all. The mental state it produces is quite unpleasant and it has little to recommend it as a "trip" unless a very low dose is used under just the right circumstances.

At this time we do not know the mechanism of action of this drug. Also, we don't know its therapeutic safety ratio. It is too new a drug. However, I rather doubt that something that causes as unpleasant an experience as phencyclidine will really catch on.

There are a number of other chemicals that can cause bizarre mental effects when taken at a very high dose. For that matter, almost any stimulant compound, including caffeine, can cause hallucinations and bizarre behavior if too much is taken. However, these chemicals are seldom deliberately used as hallucinogens. They are of academic interest only, except in poisoning cases. The world is full of hallucinogenic drugs. Anywhere you go you can get a trip, if you wish, by using some exotic native drug, for example, the plants of the Ibogaine family in Africa, in the Polynesian Islands, kava, and in New Guinea, the fish that cause bizarre mental experiences when eaten. If we can judge from past history, there will always be a certain number of people who will seek new, bizarre mental experiences by the use of chemical agents — no matter what the risk.

Marijuana

The use of marijuana in Abyssinia occurred as early as 500 B.C. Its use has spread all over the world, both as a means of pleasure and relaxation and as an important ingredient in folk medicine. It has been used by hundreds upon hundreds of millions of people over the centuries. It is estimated that marijuana is used by two hundred million people in the world right now. Its use in the United States is a relatively recent phenomenon. Marijuana was first introduced in the United States by groups of migrant workers coming into the south and southwest United States from Mexico. Through the 1930s, the drug was associated with people of lower socio-economic status. Thus, it came to have a very bad reputation, not so much from the actions of the drug, but from its association with kinds of people our society looked down on. This was the source of much of the mythology that still permeates the atmosphere surrounding marijuana. Highly placed officials proclaimed that marijuana was a "killer weed" that led its user to violent crime, insanity, sexual promiscuity, and death. Anecdotes abounded, solid data were ignored. Since this time, however, with the recent increase in the use of the drug, opinions have been changing. It is now estimated that twenty-eight million Americans have tried the drug at least once; many have continued to use marijuana on an intermittent basis. It is absolutely necessary for us to increase our understanding of this particular drug.

The discussion of a subject as controversial as marijuana is complex. The use of marijuana is enmeshed with our entire social picture. Its action as a drug cannot be separated from its sociological significance. However, the purpose of this book is not to provide a sociological analysis but to try to describe what drugs are and how they work. Therefore, for those who are interested in an authoritative report on the entire marijuana question, from its chemical effects to its sociological consequences, its relation to crime, or its use being treated as a crime, I would suggest you purchase the book *Marijuana: A Symbol of Misunderstanding: A Report of the National Commission on Marijuana and Drug Abuse* from the Superintendent of Documents, US Government Printing Office, Washington, D.C., 20402, for one dollar. This report was completed in March 1972. It presents a carefully reasoned, accurate picture of the entire marijuana question in understandable language. It was prepared by a very distinguished commission appointed by the President and Congress of the United States.

Marijuana (pot, grass, Mary Jane, MJ) is a natural product composed of the (active) flowers and top leaves and also (inactive) stalk and seeds, of the plant cannabis indica, or cannabis sativa. Various other preparations of this drug are also available, such as hashish (hash), which is the enriched form of marijuana in which more of the active resinous substance excreted from this plant is present. You might think of the relationship of marijuana to hashish being the same as that of beer to whiskey. The active chemical is the same, but one form is much more potent than its counterpart. Various other types of preparations of cannabis are found in different parts of the world. It is known by different names in different countries. A brief, partial listing of these includes kef, bhang, charas, and ganja. Each of these cannabis products varies in its content of the active chemical.

The active chemical that causes the mental effects of all cannabis products is tetrahydrocannabinol (THC). In American marijuana, the tetrahydrocannabinol content is generally less than 1 percent. On the other hand, marijuana coming from Jamaica or Southeast Asia can have as high as 2 to 4 percent THC content. Hashish generally contains between 5 and 12 percent THC.

The average dose of marijuana consumed varies between one-half of a cigarette to five to seven cigarettes at one sitting. The effects of the drug will be dependent upon the usual factors that we have already discussed: the sensitivity of the person to the drug, the amount of active chemical consumed, the frequency with which he consumes the drug, what he expects from the drug, and the setting in which the drug use takes place.

Users of marijuana can generally be classified as experimenters, they have used it a few times; intermittent users, once or twice a week; very heavy, chronic users who take five to seven cigarettes of marijuana or use hashish every day for a lifetime. Usage patterns in the United States almost entirely involve experimenters, with some of these becoming intermittent users. Also, in the United States, marijuana is usually consumed in a group. It is a group experience

— a social drug use. However, occasionally, some very heavy users do smoke by themselves. This is the rare case, not the usual drug use pattern in the United States at this time.

The immediate effects of marijuana are a slight increase in heart rate, up to about one hundred ten beats per minute, and a reddening of the eyes. If a person smokes the drug so it enters his body through his lungs it starts its action in just a few minutes. The person will generally experience the effect for a period of between half an hour and two or three hours. The state is characterized by a feeling of well-being and a heightened sensitivity to sensation, particularly taste. Foods taste delicious under marijuana, which, by the way, often leads to weight gains in marijuana users. The user seems to feel that he understands people better, and he likes people better. There is an enhancement in sensitivity to colors and forms as well as an increase of sociability. In the vast majority of cases, these sensations are described as pleasant by people who have experienced them. Following the relaxed feeling of well-being and enhanced sensory sensitivity, the person generally drifts into sleep. The sleep is usually characterized by an increase in pleasant dreams. These are the effects that would be expected from the consumption of from one-half to three or four cigarettes by the average, intermittent marijuana user who is not overly sensitive to the drug.

Observations of volunteer research subjects taking marijuana have shown that the drug can produce disconnected thought processes. The subject is often unaware that his thinking is impaired. Some students find marijuana use interferes with their ability to concentrate on their studies. Some psychiatric patients find their symptoms are aggravated by marijuana use. Although these bad effects of marijuana are not experienced by everyone, they do occur. As with any drug, undesirable effects can be a problem with marijuana.

Overuse of a drug with pleasurable effects is often indulged in by people who have problems, and this makes it difficult to tell whether using the drug is causing maladjustment or is a result of maladjustment. This complicated situation is responsible for much of our present concern over the use of drugs such as marijuana. Alcohol presents a similar set of problems.

A few people have a high degree of sensitivity to the drug. For these people or if a person has taken a very large dose, adequate to yield approximately 35 mg to 40 mg of pure THC (this is almost impossible to achieve by smoking American marijuana cigarettes), there may be a reaction in which perceptual distortion takes place. This is similar to a mild LSD experience. However, this is a relatively rare phenomenon. It takes quite a bit of drug, far beyond the usual amount taken by the intermittent, or even heavy, user. Similarly, on occasion, if the circumstances are quite unfavorable or a person is not in the right mood or was talked into "turning on," the experience can go sour. Often older people aren't prepared for the experience. They expect to "turn off," as with alcohol, rather than have an increase of awareness and sensitivity. These older people will sometimes have a mild panic reaction to marijuana. However, these panic reactions go away within a few hours, unless other people in the environment also start to panic. This agitation by others tends to make the panic reaction worse. To repeat, panic reactions are a phenomenon of those who are novices or people who are not prepared for the experience by a warm, sheltering group. It almost never occurs in an experienced user.

Very rarely, a psychotic episode can result from ingestion of cannabis products, usually hashish or the more potent of the compounds. The exact likelihood of psychotic episodes is not known but it certainly seems to be well below 0.5 percent of all users.

At this time, no proven case of lethality due to an acute overdose of marijuana is known. Animal studies make us believe that the therapeutic safety ratio is exceedingly large, perhaps 1:10,000 or more. There is no evidence to support the position that marijuana leads to increased crime, except insofar as marijuana use itself is a crime. There is no evidence, at this time, to support the belief that intermittent or moderate use of the drug, even for prolonged periods, such as ten years, leads to any changes in personality or to any alteration in the degree of social participation by the users.

They work, get married, and so on, just like everybody else. There is no evidence, at this time, to show any degree of physical dependence on the drug. However, since marijuana produces a state people enjoy, one can say that there is a psychic dependence. People do seek to obtain marijuana to try to have this pleasant experience more than once. At the present time, there is no evidence to suggest that marijuana per se, in intermittent or moderate usage, leads directly to, or causes, the use of other drugs. If there is any evidence of increased use of other drugs, those drugs seem to be tobacco and alcohol. People who smoke marijuana tend to have a higher percentage of use of tobacco and alcohol. If one is involved with people who use marijuana as an illegal drug, they then have access to other illegal drugs. Therefore, a certain percentage of people who use marijuana may try other illegal drugs also. However, not many do.

The prolonged, heavy use of marijuana, and by this I mean the daily use of six to seven cigarettes for ten years or more, does seem to be associated with a tendency toward malnutrition and a dropping out from society. It should be stressed that this is a rare phenomenon in the United States; probably less than 1 percent of all marijuana users will ever go into this steady, prolonged usage. We don't know whether the drug causes the dropping out from society, or whether society has caused the dropping out and with it some associated drug use. This is a very difficult question to answer. On the whole, however, I think I can safely state that as a public health problem, or indeed, as a problem in terms of the future strength, values, and morality of our society, the use of marijuana, per se, is of trivial importance, since it doesn't seem to be too hazardous in the way it is usually used.

I am inclined to regard the physiological and psychological effects of the social prohibitions of the drug, that is, being called a criminal and sent to jail, as far more important than the physiological and psychological effects of the drug use itself. We have no evidence that causes us to believe that the use of marijuana produces a public health problem. On the other hand, jail can cause an awful physiological and psychological effect.

An interesting new finding is that the active principle of marijuana can be used to reduce the nausea and discomfort following cancer treatments. Its medical use for this will probably soon be approved.

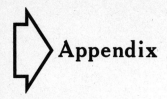

Appendix

Drug Names

Generic names are in order of mention in text. Not all proprietary names are listed for each drug and some are compounds in which the generic drug is included.

▶ Chapter 3
Sleeping Pills

GENERIC NAME	PROPRIETARY NAMES
chloral hydrate	Noctec Aquachloral Felsules
trichloroethanol	None
petrichloral	Perichlor
chloral betaine	Beta-Chlor
trichloroethylphosphate	Triclos

GENERIC NAME	PROPRIETARY NAMES
chlorobutanol	Chloretone
thiopental	Pentothal
amobarbital	Amytal In: Dexamyl, Tuinal
aprobarbital	Alurate In: Qui-A-Zone
butabarbital	Butisol In: Coastalgesic, Butibel, Plexonal
pentobarbital	Nembutal In: Emesert, Matropinal Forte, Nebralin, Stopp
secobarbital	Seconal In: Antora-B, Corovas, Gaysal, Seco-8
vinbarbital	Delvinal
phenobarbital	Luminal In: Donnatal, Belap, Antrocol, Arco-Lase Plus, Bar-Tropin, Bentyl, Bronkolixir, Bronkotab, Cantil, Chardonna, Donphen, Duotrate, Eskabarb, Gaysal, Gustase, Homapin, Isordil, Levsin, Levsinex, Lubylin, Matropinal, Mudrane, Oxoids, Pamine, Peritrate, Phazyme PB, Probital, Quadrinal, Qui-A-Zone, S.B.P., Sedadrops, Solfoton, Tensodin, Verequad, and others
mephobarbital	Mebaral, Mebroin
metharbital	Gemonil
glutethimide	Doriden
ethinamate	Valmid

GENERIC NAME	PROPRIETARY NAMES
methyprylon	Noludar
methaqualone	Quaalude, Sopor, Parest
ethchlorvynol	Placidyl
nitrazepam	Mogadon
oxazepam	Serax
flurazepam	Dalmane
scopolamine or hyoscyamine	Is found in almost all over-the-counter sleep preparations
methapyrilene	Is found in Allerest, Cope, Excedrin, Histadyl, Matropinal, Citra, Citra Forte, Co-Pyronil, Dri-Toxen, Hista-Clopane, and many others
pyrilamine maleate	Is found in Citra, Codimal, Duadacin, Eme-Nil, Emesert, Fiogesic, 4-Way Nasal Spray, Histalet, Hycomine, Matropinal Forte, Napril, Stopp, Triaminic, Tussagesic, Tussaminic, Ursinus, WANS
hydroxyzine	Atarax, Ataraxoid, Cartrax, Enarax, Marax, Vistaril, Vistrax
doxylamine	Bendectin

▶ Chapter 4
Antiseptics

Most antiseptics are in preparations. For the most part, you must look at the ingredients label, which will specify the various generic names of the drugs. Accordingly, only a few of the drugs that have specific proprietary names will be mentioned here.

GENERIC NAME	PROPRIETARY NAMES
phenol	Bakers P&S, Chloraseptic, Oraderm
hexachlorophene	Bensulfoid, pHisoHex, Soy-Dome
boric acid	Onycho-Phytex, Trimo-San
nitromersol	Butyn Metaphen
phenylmercuric acetate	Lorophyn, Nylmerate, Trimo-San
thimerosal	Merthiolate
merbromin	Mercurochrome

▶ Chapter 5
Stimulants

GENERIC NAME	PROPRIETARY NAMES
methylamphetamine	Syndrox, Norodin, Desoxyn, Fetamin
amphetamine	Dexedrine, Benzedrine, Delcobese, Fetamin, Obetrol, Biphetamine
phenmetrazine	Preludin
benzphetamine	Didrex
phentermine	Fastin, Ionamin
diethylpropion	Tenuate, Tepanil
phendimetrazine	Bacarate, Bontril, Melfiat, Obe-nil, Plegine, Statobex, Trimstat, Trimtabs
methylphenidate	Ritalin

▶ Chapter 6
Stomach Drugs

The following stomach drugs do not have proprietary names

sodium bicarbonate

calcium carbonate

magnesium trisalicylate

dihydroxy aluminum amino-acetate

magnesium carbonate

charcoal

bismuth subcarbonate

bismuth subnitrate

kaolin

pectin

aluminum hydroxide

homatropine

atropine methyl nitrate

atropine sulfate

castor oil

phenolphthalein

cascara sagrada

magnesium citrate

sodium phosphate

potassium phosphate

methylcellulose

sodium carboxymethyl cellulose

tragacanth

bran

mineral oil

Stomach Drugs with Proprietary Names

GENERIC NAME	PROPRIETARY NAMES
magnesium hydroxide	Milk of Magnesia
scopolamine	Dolonil, Donphen, Sidonna
methantheline	Banthine
propantheline	Pro-Banthine, Probital
oxyphenonium	Antrenyl
anisotropine	Valpin
diphemanil	Prantal
glycopyrrolate	Robinul
hexocyclium	Tral
isopropamide	Darbid
mepenzolate	Cantil
pipenzolate	Piptal

GENERIC NAME	PROPRIETARY NAMES
poldine	Nacton
tridihexethyl	Pathilon, Milpath
cyclandelate	Cyclospasmol
oxyphencyclimine	Daricon, Vio-thene
piperidolate	Dactil
clidinium	Librax
thiphenamil	Trocinate
adiphenine	Trasentine
dicyclomine	Bentyl, Dyspas, Bendectin
dimenhydrinate	Dramamine
cyclizine	Marezine
meclizine	Bonine, Antivert
trimethobenzamide	Tigan
chlorpromazine	Thorazine
promethazine	Allergan, Phenergan, Mepergan
meprobamate	Equanil, Miltown
bisacodyl	Dulcolax, Bicol
magnesium sulfate	Epsom salts
sodium sulfate	Glaubers salt
potassium sodium tartrate	Rochelle salt
psyllium	Plantago

GENERIC NAME	PROPRIETARY NAMES
dioctyl sodium sulfosuccinate	Colace, Doxinate, and many others
poloxysocol	Magsol, Polycol
diphenoxylate	Lomotil

▷ Chapter 7
Analgesics

GENERIC NAME	PROPRIETARY NAMES
aspirin	In almost every pain relieving mixture
phenacetin	Buff-A-Comp, Empirin, Emprazil, Fiorinal, Metrogesics, Phenaphen, Soma, Synalgos
acetaminophen	Datril, Excedrin, Sinarest, Tempra, Trinol, Tylenol, Sinutab, Vanquish, and many others
The local anesthetics xylocaine, dibucaine, and benzocaine are in numerous lotions, sprays, lozenges, etc.	
oxycodone	Percodan
meperidine	Demerol
methadone	Dolophine, Amidone, Methenex
dextromethorphan	Is in most cough remedies
diphenoxylate	Lomotil
ethoheptazine	Zactirin
propoxyphene	Darvon

GENERIC NAME	PROPRIETARY NAMES
pentazocine	Talwin
ergotamine	Gynergen, Ergomar
ergotamine and caffeine	Cafergot, Migral
colchicine	ColBenemid
allopurinol	Zyloprim
probenecid	Benemid
phenylbutazone	Butazolidin, Azolid
oxyphenbutazone	Tandearil, Oxalid
indomethacin	Indocin

▶ Chapter 8
Hormones

GENERIC NAME	PROPRIETARY NAMES
diethylstilbestrol	Acnestrol, Tylosterone
ethinyl estradiol	In: Android-G, Brevicon, Demulen, Estinyl, Feminone, Gevrine, Gynetone, Haldorin, Loestrin, Lo/Ovral, Norlestrin, Oracon, Os-Cal, Ovral, Testand, Test-Estrin, Zorane
mestranol	Demulen, Estinyl, Loestrin, Norlestrin, Ovral
conjugated estrogen	Evex, Premarin
chlorotrianisene	Tace
progesterone	Duphaston, Proluton

GENERIC NAME	PROPRIETARY NAMES
medroxyprogesterone	Provera
hydroxyprogesterone	Delalutin
norethindrone	Norinyl, Norlestrin, Ortho-Novum
insulin	Iletin
tolbutamide	Orinase
acetohexamide	Dymelor
tolazamide	Tolinase
chlorpropamide	Diabinese
phenformin	Meltrol
hydrocortisone	There are over 100 different compounds with this ingredient listed on the label
prednisolone	Ataraxoid, Delta-Cortef, Meticortelone, Meti-Derm, Sterapred, Metimyd, Neo-Delta-Cortef, Sterane, Metreton, Opti-myd
prednisone	Betapar, Delta-Dome, Deltasone, Meti-corten, Orasone, Sterapred, Sterazoli-din
triamcinolone	Aristocort, Kenacort, Kenalog, Mycolog, Aristospan
paramethasone	Haldrone
betamethasone	Benisone, Celestone, Flurobate, Dipro-sone, Valisone
dexamethasone	Aeroseb-Dex, Decaderm, Decadron, De-ronil, Dexone, Gammacorten, Hexadrol

GENERIC NAME	PROPRIETARY NAMES
thyroid	Cytomel, Euthroid, Letter, Proloid, S-P-T, Synthroid, Thyroid, Thyrolar
thyroxine	Choloxin, Cytolen, Levoid
propylthiouracil	None
methylthiouracil	Methiacil, Thimecil
carbimazole	Neomercazole

▶ Chapter 9
Tranquilizers, Muscle Relaxants, and Anticonvulsives

GENERIC NAME	PROPRIETARY NAMES
chlorpromazine	Thorazine, Largactil, Megaphen, Chlor-P2
haloperidol	Haldol
benztropine mesylate	Cogentin
trihexyphenidyl	Artane, Pipanol, Tremin
promazine	Sparine
triflupromazine	Vesprin
fluphenazine	Permitil
fluphenazine enanthate or fluphenazine decanoate	Prolixin
perphenazine	Trilafon, Triavil, Etrafon
prochlorperazine maleate	Compazine Maleate
prochlorperazine edisylate	Compazine Edisylate

GENERIC NAME	PROPRIETARY NAMES
trifluoperazine	Stelazine
thioridazine	Mellaril
acetophenazine	Tindal
promethazine	Phenergan, Quadnite, Synalgos, Zipan-25
chlorprothixene	Taractan
thiothixene	Navane
reserpine	Serpasil
meprobamate	Miltown, Equanil, PMB-200, PMB-400, Pathibamate, QID-Bamate, SK-Bamate
tybamate	Solacen, Tybatran
carisoprodol	Rela, Soma
mebutamate	Capla
hydoxyphenamate	Listica
ethinamate	Valmid
buclizine	Bucladin-S
hydroxyzine	Atarax, Ataraxiod, Cartrax, Enarax, Marax, Vistaril, Vistrax
chlordiazepoxide	Librium, Menrium, Libritabs, Librax
diazepam	Valium
clorazepate	Tranxene
oxazepam	Serax

GENERIC NAME	PROPRIETARY NAMES
doxepin	Sinequan, Adapin
methocarbamol	Robaxin, Robaxisal
styramate	Sinaxar
chlorzoxazone	Paraflex, Parafon
phenobarbital	Luminal (In many compounds)
metharbital	Gemonil
mephobarbital	Mebaral, Mebroin
primidone	Mysoline
diphenylhydantoin	Dilantin, Diphenyl, Ekko
mephenytoin	Mesantoin
phenylethylhydantoin	Nirvanol
ethotoin	Peganone
albutoin	Co-ord
phenacemide	Phenurone
trimethadione	Tridione
paramethadione	Paradione
phensuximide	Milontin
methsuximide	Celontin
ethosuximide	Zarontin

GENERIC NAME	PROPRIETARY NAMES
sulfanilamide	Prontosil, AVC, Sulfamal, Vagitrol
sulfacytine	Renoquid
sulfadiazine	Quinette, Suladyne, Benegyn
sulfabenzamide	Sultrin
sulfamethizole	Azotrex, Suladyne, Thiosulfil, Urobiotic
sulfacetamide	Sultrin
sulfasalazine	Azulfidine, Rorasul, SAS-500
sulfamethazine	Octin
sulfisoxazole	Gantrisin, Azo-Gantrisin, SK-Soxazole, Soxomide, Vagilia
sulfamethoxazole	Gantanol, Azo Gantanol, Bactrim, Septra
sulfamethoxypyridazine	Midicel
sulfadimethoxine	Madribon
sulfameter	Sulla
penicillin G	Crysticillin, Depo-Penicillin, Diurnal-Penicillin, Lentopen, Bicillin, Duracillin, Pentids, Pfizerpen G, QID pen G, Wycillin
phenethicillin	Darcil, Chemipen, Maxipen, Syncillin
methicillin	Staphcillin, Celbenin

GENERIC NAME	PROPRIETARY NAMES
amoxicillin	Amoxil, Larotid, Polymox
oxacillin	Prostaphlin, Bactocill
cloxacillin	Orbenin, Tegopen
dicloxacillin	Dynapen, Pathocil, Veracillin
nafcillin	Unipen
ampicillin	Amcill, Omnipen, Pen-A, Penbritin, Poly-cillin, Principen, Pensyn, QID amp, Supen
hetacillin	Penplenum, Versapen
carbenicillin	Geocillin
phenoxymethyl penicillin	Potassium Penicillin V, Compocillin-VK, Pen-Vee K, V-Cillin K, Betapen-VK, Veetids, Pfizerpen VK, Robicillin VK, QUID pen VK, Uticillin VK, SK-Peni-cillin VK
probenecid	Benemid, ColBENEMID
streptomycin	None
chloramphenicol	Chloromycetin
tetracyclines	Aureomycin, Terramycin, Achromycin, Declomycin, Minocin, Vibramycin, Panmycin, QID tet, Robitet, Sumycin, Retet
isoniazid	INH, Nydrazid
cycloserine	Seromycin
para-aminosalicylic acid	PAS
viomycin	Viocin

317 ◀◀◀

GENERIC NAME	PROPRIETARY NAMES
ethambutol	Myambutol
rifampin	Rifadin, Rifamate, Rimactane, Rimactazid
erythromycin	Ilotycin, Erythrocin, Pediamycin, Bristamycin, Robimycin Ethril, QID mycin, E-mycin
cephalothin	Keflin
cephaloridine	Loridine
cephaloglycin	Kafocin
neomycin	Mycifradin, Myciguent. In many creams, ointments, etc.
paromycin	Humatin
kanamycin	Kantrex
polymyxin B	Aerosporin, Biotres, Lidosporin, Neo-Polycin, Neosporin, Polycin, Polysporin, Otobione Otocort, Cortisporin
colistin	Coly-Mycin
vancomycin	Vancocin
cephalexin	Keflex
cephapirin	Cafadyl
cephradine	Anspor, Velosef
bacitracin	Found in many ointments and sprays
lincomycin	Lincocin
gentamicin	Garamycin

GENERIC NAME	PROPRIETARY NAMES
nystatin	Mycostatin, Achrostatin, Declostatin, Florotic, Korostatin, Mycolog, Nilstat, Nystaform, Terrastatin
amphotericin B	Fungizone, Mysteclin-F
griseofulvin	Fulvicin, Grifulvin, Grisactin, Gris-Peg
tolnaftate	Tinactin
undecylenic acid	In many foot powders

▶ Chapter 11
Antidepressants

GENERIC NAME	PROPRIETARY NAMES
Imipramine	Trofranil, Imavate, Janimine, Presamine, SK-Pramine
desmethylimipramine	Norpramin, Pertofrane
amitriptyline	Elavil, Etrafon, Triavil
northriptyline	Aventyl
protriptyline	Vivactil
Lithium	Eskalith, Lithane, Lithonate, Lithotabs, Pfi-Lithium

▶ Chapter 12
Shotgun Cold Remedies

There are so many different cold remedies on the market, it is almost impossible to list them all. Look at the label to see the composition of the particular mixture. Listed are just a few proprietary names.

GENERIC NAME	PROPRIETARY NAMES
diphenhydramine	Benadryl, Benylin
carbinoxamine	Clistin, Rondec

GENERIC NAME	PROPRIETARY NAMES
tripelennamine	Pyribenzamine, Rhulihist
pyrilamine	Neo-Antergan, Copsamine, Paraminyl, Thylogen, and many others
antazoline	Antistine
methapyrilene	Dozar, Histadyl, Buffadyne, Thenylene, Cope, and many others
cyproheptadine	Periactin
chlorpheniramine	Chlor-Trimeton, Teldrin, Antagonate, Histaspan, and many others
dexbrompheniramine	Dimetane, Disomer, Drixoral
dexchlorpheniramine	Polaramine
chlorcyclizine	Fedrazil, Mantadil
triprolidine	Actidil, Actifed
phenylephrine	Neo-Synephrine, Isophrine, Azolid, and many others
hydroxyamphetamine	Paredrine
naphazoline	Pyribine, 4-Way Nasal Spray, Privine
tetrahydrozoline	Tyzine, Visine
oxymetazoline	Afrin
xylometazoline	Otrivin
cyclopentamine	Clopane, Aerolone, Co-Pyronil
phenylpropanolamine	Allerest, Coricidin and many others, including hunger reducing preparations
propylhexedrine	Benzedrex

GENERIC NAME	PROPRIETARY NAMES
tuaminoheptane	None
ephedrine	Tedral, Mudrane, Verequad, Ectasule, Isuprel, Rynatuss, Bronkotabs, and others

▶ Chapter 13
Vitamins and Minerals

No listing of vitamin or mineral preparations is included. Look on the package to see what vitamins and minerals are in a given preparation. Then compare the amounts to your needs.

▶ Chapter 14
Drugs for the Skin

No listing of individual drugs will be included since there is an almost infinite set of combinations on the market.

▶ Chapter 15
Drugs and the Kidneys

GENERIC NAME	PROPRIETARY NAMES
chlorothiazide	Diuril, Aldoclor, Diupres
hydrochlorothiazide	Hydrodiuril, Esidrix, Aldactazide, Aldoril, Butiserpazide, Butizide, Dyazide, Esimil, Hydropres, Hydrotensin, Hydro-Z-50, Lexxor, Oretic, Oreticyl, Ser-Ap-Es, Unipres
bendroflumethiazide	Naturetin, Rauzide
benzthiazide	Exna, Aquatag
polythiazide	Renese

GENERIC NAME	PROPRIETARY NAMES
cyclothiazide	Anhydron
methyclothiazide	Enduron, Aquatensen, Diutensin, Enduronyl, Eutron
trichlormethiazide	Naqua, Metahydrin, Metatensin, Naquival
merbaphen	Novasurol
mersalyl	Salyrgan
acetazolamide	Diamox
ethacrynic acid	Edecrin
furosemide	Lasix
spironolactone	Aldactone, Aldactazide
triamterene	Dyrenium, Dyazide

▶ Chapter 16
Drugs for the Heart

GENERIC NAME	PROPRIETARY NAMES
digitalis	Crystodigin
digoxin	Lanoxin
ouabain	Strophanthin-G
lanatoside C	Cedilanid
deslanoside	Cedilanid-D
acetyldigitoxin	Acylanid
gitalin	Gitaligin

GENERIC NAME	PROPRIETARY NAMES
quinidine	Quinamin, Quinaglute, Cardioquin, Quinidex, Quinora
propranolol	Inderal
nitrates and nitrites	Amyl nitrite, Antora, Iso-Bid, Nitrol, Nitrong, Pentritol, Peritrate, Sorbide
nitroglycerin	Nitrol, Nitro-Bid, Nitroglyn, Nitrong, Nitrospan, Nitrostat
erythrityl tetranitrate	Cardilate
isosorbide dinitrate	Isordil, Iso-Bid, Laserdil, Sorbide, Sorbitrate
mannitol hexanitrate	None
trolnitrate	None
pentaerythritol tetranitrate	Antora, Cartrax, Corovas, Duotrate, Miltrate, Papavatral, Pentritol, Peritrate, SK-Petn
reserpine	Serpasil, Butiserpazide, Diupres, Diutensen, Dralserp, Exna-R, Hydromox, Hydropres, Hydrotensin, Metatensin, Naquival, Rau-Sed, Regroton, Renese-R, Salutensin, Sandril, Ser-Ap-Es
methyldopa	Aldomet, Aldoclor, Aldoril
hydralazine	Apresoline, Dralserp, Dralzine, Hydrotensin Plus, Ser-Ap-Es, Unipres
guanethidine	Ismelin, Esimil

▶ **Chapter 17**
Hallucinogens and Marijuana

No proprietary names are listed.

Bibliography

The following are books your physician may use and upon which I leaned heavily in writing this book:

Goodman, L., and Gilman, A., eds. *The Pharmacological Basis of Therapeutics.* 5th ed. New York: Macmillan, 1975.
Merck Manual of Diagnosis and Therapy, The. 13th ed., edited by R. Berkow. Rahway, N.J.: Merck & Co., 1977.
Physician's Desk Reference, The. 29th ed., edited by C. E. Baker. Oradell, N.J.: Litton Publications, Medical Economics, 1977.

Books written for the nonprofessional:

Burack, R. *The New Handbook of Prescription Drugs.* New York: Ballantine Books, 1970.
Handbook of Non-Prescription Drugs, The. Edited by G. Griffenhagen and E. Hawkins. American Pharmaceutical Association, 1971.
Interim Report of the Commission of Inquiry into the Non-Medical Use of Drugs. G. LeDain, Chairman, Queen's Printer, 1970.
Long, J. W. *The Essential Guide to Prescription Drugs.* New York: Harper & Row, 1977.
U.S. Government Printing Office. *Marijuana: A Signal of Misunderstanding.* Washington, D.C.: Government Printing Office, R. P. Shafer, Chairman, 1972.

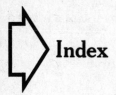

Index

Lasix, 266
Lauryl ether, 258
Lauryl isoquinoline bromide, 254
Laurylic acid, 254
Laxatives, 97–102; bulk-forming, 99–100; cathartic, 97–98; dependence on, 102; emollient, 100–102; saline, 98–99
Lentopen, 188
Librax, 93
Librium, 161–162
Licorice root, 248
Lidocaine, 114
Lincocin, 196
Lincomycin, 196
Listica, 161
Lithium, 208–209
Loestrin, 133
Lomotil, 124, 103
Loridine, 195–196
Lorophyn, 70
LSD. *See* Lysergic acid diethylamide
Luminal, 52
Lyndiol, 134
Lysergic acid diethylamide, 283–290

MA. *See* Amphetamines
Macrodantin, 73
Madribon, 183
Magnesium carbonate, 89, 97, 99
Magnesium citrate, 97, 99
Magnesium hydroxide, 89, 97, 99
Magnesium oxide, 97, 99
Magnesium stearate, 250
Magnesium sulfate, 97, 98
Magnesium trisilicate, 89, 92–93
Magsol, 101
Mania, 208–209
Mannitol, 265
Mannitol hexanitrate, 275
Marezine, 95, 216
Marijuana, 295–301
Mary Jane. *See* Marijuana
Maxipen, 188
MDA. *See* Amphetamines
Measures, drug, 22
Mebaral, 52, 169
Mebutamate, 161
Meclizine, 92, 216
Meclizine hydrochloride, 95
Meditrol, 83

Medrol, 144–145
Medroxyprogesterone, 133
Megavitamin therapy, 241
Mellaril, 157
Meltrol, 141–142
Menopause, 132
Menstruation, 131–132
Menthol, 113, 258
Mepenzolate, 93
Mepergan, 96
Meperidine, 117–120
Mephenytoin, 170
Mephobarbital, 52
Meprobamate, 92, 96, 158–160, 165
Merbaphen, 266
Merbromin, 70
Mercuric chloride, 70
Mercurochrome, 70
Mercury bichloride, 70
Mercury chloride, 102
Mercury diuretics, 266
Mercury ointment, 70
Mersalyl, 266
Merthiolate, 70
Mesantoin, 170
Mescaline, 290–293
Mestranol, 133
Metal salt antiseptics, 70–71
Metaphen, 70
Methacoline chloride, 113
Methadone, 117–119, 123–124
Methantheline, 95
Methantheline bromide, 93
Methapyrilene, 58, 215
Metharbital, 52, 169
Methaqualone, 55
Methenex, 118–119
Methicillin, 188
Methocarbamol, 164
Methoxyamphetamine, 291
Methoxymethyleneoxyamphetamine, 291
Methsuximide, 172
Methyclothiazide, 265
Methyl salicylate, 113
Methylamphetamine, 81, 83–84
Methylbenzethonium chloride, 72, 252
Methylcellulose, 97, 100, 248
Methyldopa, 277
Methylenedioxyamphetamine, 291
Methylthiouracil, 150